HEART
Solution
for
WOMEN

A Proven Program to Prevent and
Reverse Heart Disease

MARK MENOLASCINO
MD, MS, ABIHM, ABAARM, IFMCP

Founder and Medical Director of
The Meno Clinic Center for Functional Medicine

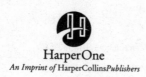

HarperOne
An Imprint of HarperCollins*Publishers*

HarperOne

This book contains advice and information relating to health care. It should be used to supplement rather than replace the advice of your doctor or another trained health professional. If you know or suspect you have a health problem, it is recommended that you seek your physician's advice before embarking on any medical program or treatment. All efforts have been made to assure the accuracy of the information contained in this book as of the date of publication. This publisher and the author disclaim liability for any medical outcomes that may occur as a result of applying the methods suggested in this book.

FIRST EDITION

Designed by SBI Book Arts, LLC

Library of Congress Cataloging-in-Publication Data

Names: Menolascino, Mark, author.
Title: Heart solution for women : a proven program to prevent and reverse heart disease / Mark Menolascino, MD, MS, ABIHM, ABAARM, IFMCP, founder and Medical Director of The Meno Clinic-Center for Functional Medicine.
Description: First edition. | [San Francisco, California] : HarperOne, [2019] | Includes bibliographical references and index.
Identifiers: LCCN 2018040470 (print) | LCCN 2018052981 (ebook) | ISBN 9780062842169 (e-book) | ISBN 9780062842138 | ISBN 9780062842138(hardcover) | ISBN 9780062842145(paperback) | ISBN 9780062864895(audio)
Subjects: LCSH: Heart diseases in women—Prevention. | Heart diseases in women—Alternative treatment.
Classification: LCC RC682 (ebook) | LCC RC682 .M46 2019 (print) | DDC 616.1/20082—dc23
LC record available at https://lccn.loc.gov/2018040470

19 20 21 22 23 LSC 10 9 8 7 6 5 4 3 2 1

To my loving children,
Anthony Fisher and Jueliet Jade.
You brighten all my days and fill my heart with love
I am so proud of you both.

Contents

Foreword

As a personalized nutrition physician and weight-loss specialist, I've spent my entire career talking to women about their health. Through my experience listening to and caring for women, one thing I know for sure is this: Ask women about their biggest health concerns, and they'll tell you they're afraid of getting breast cancer, developing diabetes, or having a stroke. But here's what most of them don't consider: *Heart disease is the #1 killer of women, and more women suffer from heart disease than all of these other conditions combined.* In fact, one in four women will develop the disease.

So why aren't women more concerned about their heart health? That's because many women, and even many of their doctors, continue to think of heart disease primarily as a "male" disease, despite the fact that heart attack rates are dropping in middle-aged men and are currently *rising* in middle-aged women.

And here's another fact: Nearly all treatments for heart disease are based on scientific research done on men, not women. This is a key reason why women who develop heart disease typically have worse outcomes than men.

If these facts alarm you, they should.

I'm writing to you, reader, to introduce my brilliant friend and colleague, Dr. Mark Menolascino, and to say thank you for picking up this important book and taking this first huge step toward preserving and protecting your heart. Dr. Menolascino, one of the most brilliant and talented medical professionals I've been honored to meet in my career, is on a mission to change these grim statistics for women. With four board certifications, Dr. Menolascino has been on the front lines of heart health and research for most of his life, running a state-of-the-art clinic where he takes a holistic approach to reversing disease and jump-starting health.

In *Heart Solution for Women*, Dr. Menolascino describes the surprising physiological differences between men's and women's hearts. He also explains how heart disease manifests differently in women than in men, creating symptoms including depression, anxiety, panic attacks, poor sleep, and chronic pain. In addition, he discusses how the symptoms of heart disease can be masked by pregnancy or post-pregnancy, only to emerge with a vengeance later in life when a woman's "heart attack advantage" disappears.

In these pages, you'll discover why women's heart disease symptoms often go overlooked for years, and why even ER doctors can fail to diagnose women's heart attacks. You'll also learn about the factors that put you at risk for heart disease—not just the well-known factors such obesity and high blood pressure, but also major culprits ranging from hormone imbalances to food sensitivities to a sick gut. In addition, you'll get the facts about the dangers of current medications for heart disease (for example, did you know that statins can increase your risk of diabetes by up to 50 percent?) and find out how to minimize or stop your use of these drugs.

Finally—and most important of all—Dr. Menolascino guides you step by step through an in-depth assessment that will empower you to develop your own personalized plan for slashing your risk of heart disease or healing an already-damaged heart. This plan includes simple, doable actions such as adding heart-healing foods to your diet (like my favorite, bone broth!), taking the right supplements, and changing your exercise routine from pro-inflammatory to anti-inflammatory workouts.

Featuring the latest research on heart, gut, brain, and hormone health and including answers to the most common misunderstandings about heart health, *Heart Solution for Women* will give you all the tools you need to keep your amazing heart beating strongly for life.

—*Dr. Kellyann Petrucci*
New York Times bestselling author of *Dr. Kellyann's Bone Broth Diet* and creator of DrKellyann.com
Host of the public television special "21 Days to a Slimmer, Younger You"

Author's Note

I've spent most of my life studying the complexities of healing the human body. During my free time, I read peer-reviewed articles from respected medical journals and travel dozens of times each year to lecture at, and learn from, medical conferences all over the world. Back home in Jackson Hole, Wyoming, at the base of the spectacular Teton Mountains, I run the Meno Clinic Center for Functional Medicine. I'm one of five doctors in my family—both of my brothers are internal medicine specialists, my sister is a psychiatrist, and my father was one of the world's experts in his field. Healing the human body is in my blood, and not a day passes that I don't obsess over how to do it better.

In my search for the best medical training available, I ended up with four board certifications and a double master's degree and became a specialist in what is now called "functional medicine." This term was only recently coined, but the premise of functional medicine—treating the whole body and not just individual symptoms—is as old as medicine itself; its roots can be traced back thousands of years, and its practitioners have included many of the most visionary physicians in history. When I was a young doctor, it was called "holistic medicine." As the concept of whole-body medicine matured it became known as "integrative medicine." Today functional medicine could be defined as:

Combining the art and science of integrative, holistic medicine with cutting-edge diagnostics and individualized treatment plans that include nutritional and lifestyle advice, supplements, and pharmaceuticals to heal the individual, not just relieve symptoms.

As a young doctor, I had the chance to work under Dr. Dean Ornish as part of the team implementing his heart disease reversal program and witnessed firsthand the power of customized whole-body medicine delivered with precision accuracy to the individual through lifestyle, diet, and targeted supplements. We gave a group of men scheduled for heart surgery the option of forgoing surgery and instead healing their hearts by correcting imbalances in the rest of their bodies. It worked. The men who opted out of surgery did better in every way than those who went under the knife. The experience of delivering cutting-edge lifestyle medicine to heal the heart left me with two questions:

1. How can we do this for more people?

2. Where are the women?

Decades later, after spending every waking minute obsessing over the practice of whole-body medicine, I decided to write this book to answer these two questions and put the specific tools for preventing and reversing heart disease directly into the hands of the people who need them most. Because the reality is that, when it comes to women's hearts, we've made some of the biggest mistakes in the history of human health. It's time for a change.

—*Dr. Mark Menolascino*

Part I

The Truth About Women's Hearts

Chapter 1

Unfair to the Fairer Sex

When we consider the miracles of modern medicine, it's easy to think we've arrived. The technological wonders of intensive care have all but brought people back from the dead and allowed some of us to survive even the most horrific injuries. We now have pharmaceuticals built on a molecular level and surgeons using the world's most precise tools to maneuver inside our veins, muscles, joints, and even brains. Despite these incredible capabilities, we have not arrived. Not by a long shot.

In medical school, a professor told my class, "Fifty percent of what we're about to teach you is wrong; it's up to you to figure out which half." We've made some huge gains in medicine since then, but much of the half we had wrong is still taught in medical schools, practiced in hospitals and clinics, and pervasive in mainstream culture. In my opinion—shaped through the lessons of four board certifications, a double master's degree, and the experience of treating thousands of women for chronic ailments in my clinic, where 80 percent of patients are female—no area of modern medicine is less understood than heart health in women.

Take this story for example. Sue was scheduled to have her gall-bladder removed after three days of severe heartburn. I was the doctor on call at the time, and although the decision had already been made to do the surgery, I wanted to talk to her one last time to make sure the problem was her gallbladder before sending her under the knife. Because she was having abdominal pain and not the classic chest pain associated with heart attack, no one had checked her heart enzymes, the standard method for detecting a heart attack. Women sometimes present heart attacks differently than men: although most have pressure or pain in the chest, some women can instead experience vomiting and/or stomach, back, or jaw pain—symptoms easily confused with other, less lethal ailments.

I ordered an enzyme test for Sue, just to be sure. The result? *She had been having a heart attack for three days.* Because Sue did not present the usual symptoms, we almost sent her into the operating room for gallbladder surgery while she was having a heart attack!

Instead of removing Sue's gallbladder, we sent a tiny balloon into one of her arteries and inflated it at the point where blood flow was compromised. Unfortunately for Sue, this procedure is best performed within hours of a heart attack, not after the heart has been starved for oxygen for three days. Afterwards, a cardiologist confirmed that Sue's heart muscle was severely damaged and told her she was likely to be a "cardiac cripple" for the rest of her life.

Sue's story doesn't end there, and it even has a happy ending, but to understand the path that led her to the brink of being operated on for the wrong condition, we must look at the story of heart disease and the misunderstandings about women's heart health, which go far beyond the hospital and have become deeply ingrained in our mainstream culture. The institution of medicine has not treated women's heart health with the same care and investment as men's for a number of reasons, but two are particularly important: the history of heart disease research, and the complex relationship between female hormones and female hearts.

A Man's Disease

Men have historically been the focus of heart disease research and concern, both because it develops, on average, nearly a decade later in women than in men and because more men than women die in middle age of heart disease. These facts are partly responsible for why heart disease has seemed like less of an issue for women, going as far back as the late 1800s; indeed, at that time some physicians viewed heart disease as a "macho" way to die, a sign that the deceased had been a hardworking man. This perspective changed (somewhat) thanks to studies in the 1950s that linked heart disease with lacking fitness and nutrition—in men. For the next fifty years, that trend continued: the vast majority of heart disease research favored men. While the men were being monitored for heart health, the women's hearts were largely ignored. Even as recently as the 1980s and '90s, many landmark studies on heart disease were entirely focused on men. The Multiple Risk Factor Intervention Trial of 1982, recognized as one of the first studies to prove a link between cholesterol and heart disease, involved over 12,000 men and zero women. Appropriately perhaps, its acronym is MRFIT.

In 1991, the editor of the *New England Journal of Medicine* wrote, "Heart disease is also a woman's disease, not just a man's disease in disguise." Yet the sample for the Physicians Health Study of 1995, which found that aspirin reduced the risk of heart attack, included over 20,000 men and—you guessed it—not one single woman.

According to the American Heart Association (AHA), a total of 38 percent of heart disease research subjects have been women. Even this percentage doesn't tell the whole story, since most of the heart disease studies on women have been conducted only in recent years. Also, research attempts to treat men and women equally without actually giving both an equal shake in the lab have led to unintended consequences. A 2007 article in the *Journal of the Royal Society of Medicine* explains: "The evidence bases of medicine may be fundamentally flawed because there is an ongoing failure of research tools to include sex differences in study design and analysis. The reporting bias by which this methodology maintains creates a situation where guidelines based on the study of one sex may be generalized and applied to both."

Treating women and men equally? Good idea. Treating women's bodies the same as men's in conclusions drawn from medical research? Not so much. It is now clear that we have done a huge disservice to women and their health. Thanks to all the research into men's heart health, the rate of heart attack in men between the ages of thirty-five and fifty-four is declining. In women of the same age, however, heart attack rates are increasing, and researchers have noted a particularly alarming heart attack rate increase of more than 1 percent annually among thirty-five- to forty-four-year-old women.

The other main reason women's heart health has been overlooked for the last century is that, during the reproductive years, women have a heart health advantage over men. Women's hormones, and the more flexible physical structure of women's hearts, veins, and arteries, offer a layer of protection that reduces the occurrence of heart disease in women before menopause. Their hormones give women a little more time to heal wounds, correct imbalances, and work toward optimal function before heart disease takes hold. This advantage, however, is a double-edged sword: it also obscures the picture of a woman's heart health during her younger years. Essentially, if you are premenopausal, you may have several high-risk factors for heart disease, but thanks to the protective quality of your hormones and feminine vascular system, you (and your doctor) don't even realize it.

The protective/deceptive role of women's hormones in their heart health is a tricky concept to grasp, but think of it this way: Imagine if your female hormones protected you from gaining weight for the first half of your life, but as soon as menopause hit, the weight you could have gained during those years because of your genetics and lifestyle choices suddenly appeared all at once. It would be truly shocking and terribly unfair to wake up one day with all that weight suddenly hanging from your body. This, of course, is not what happens with weight, but it does happen with heart health: younger women need to monitor and nurture their heart health in the absence of some of the feedback mechanisms available to men, or risk arriving at menopause with a dramatic, sudden, and unexpected uptick in heart disease risk—or even the seemingly sudden appearance of the disease itself.

The Big "Duh!"

The seriousness of heart disease in women is underappreciated from the living room to the examination room and all the way to the emergency room. Scenes of men having heart attacks in movies and TV shows have trained the entire world to assess men for heart disease, and yet even our most skilled health experts may dismiss the symptoms of heart distress in women. This cultural and professional misunderstanding of women's heart health has led to some terribly unfortunate trends. To this day, women with heart disease are less likely to be tested to determine its severity and less likely to undergo procedures to unclog blocked arteries, even when they and their physicians know that their arteries are compromised. And the prognosis for a woman who has a heart attack is much worse than is typical for a man. Women between the ages of forty and fifty-nine are up to four times more likely to die from heart bypass surgery than men of the same age, and all women are twice as likely as men to die within the first few weeks of suffering a heart attack.

It is my opinion that even in the emergency room, the venue for life-saving medicine, women's heart health is not treated with the same sense of urgency as men's. Doctors are blindsided every day by the markedly different symptoms of heart disease that women present: different electrical signals, problems manifesting in different areas of the heart, and different surface symptoms of heart dysfunction. What this means for a woman experiencing a heart attack that is not accompanied by the typical symptoms is that by the time the problem is diagnosed correctly, her heart muscle has already been damaged and any procedures she undergoes will be riskier than if the problem had been detected earlier. "Time is myocardium" and

"Time is the issue for the tissue" are the mantras of the heart catheterization lab, where small balloons are inserted into arteries to open blockages. We say these mantras to remind ourselves that the more time passes before intervention, the more heart damage occurs. Too many times I have seen bad things happen to women whose symptoms were misdiagnosed or for whom intervention was delayed. This is especially disheartening (literally) when early suspicion, knowledge, and intervention could have saved the day—and their heart muscle.

On Valentine's Day, I was "coerced" into watching an episode of *Grey's Anatomy*, a wildly popular TV medical drama. On this episode, Dr. Bailey, the female chief of surgery, drops off her fireman husband at work and takes herself to a different hospital ER to be evaluated for a heart attack. She goes up to the front nursing desk and blurts out, "I am having a heart attack." This highly accomplished doctor knows that she is having a heart attack, but what happens next in the ER? They make her fill out paperwork, and then wait before being seen. When she is eventually evaluated, her tests are not conclusive. Her doctors decide that either she is experiencing something else, like heartburn or anxiety and stress, or she's just a hypochondriac doctor. So the cardiologist asks about her stress at home and at work. In the end, she has to undergo very risky open-heart surgery that almost kills her.

Of course, because this is television, Dr. Bailey lives and goes on to perform miraculous surgeries. I have seen what happens to her too many times in my career, however, and in real life there is one significant difference from the made-for-TV version: the victim usually doesn't make it out of the hospital. Men and women are not the same when it comes to heart disease—whether in how it evolves, how it presents, or how they respond to treatment.

The fictional *Grey's Anatomy* story is not far from reality. From what I've seen, if a husband and wife go into the emergency room after dinner, both of them complaining of chest discomfort, the man is likely to be given a stress test to see if he is having a heart attack and the woman is likely be diagnosed with something else—just like Dr. Bailey in

Grey's Anatomy—and given heartburn medicine to relieve stomach or gallbladder upset—just like Sue.

Starting in the 2000s, the institution of medicine finally slapped its collective forehead with its collective palm and asked: What were we thinking? Even researchers who were typically not prone to making statements about what we should or should not do began to take a stand on the issue of women's heart health. In a 2010 article titled "Gender Differences in Coronary Heart Disease," the authors stated: "The under-recognition of heart disease and differences in clinical presentation in women lead to less aggressive treatment strategies and a lower representation of women in clinical trials. Furthermore, self-awareness in women and identification of their cardiovascular risk factors needs more attention, which should result in a better prevention of cardiovascular events."

A recent study showed that between the ages of forty-five and fifty-four, more women have strokes than men. Young women with diabetes have quadruple the risk of heart attack compared to young men with diabetes. And with the recent revelations about brain disease, ailments like Alzheimer's and depression are now understood to be closely related to heart health. The fact that two-thirds of Alzheimer's and depression victims are women thus raises the question: If women were advised on heart-healthy lifestyle choices by their doctors with the same regularity as men, would fewer women suffer from depression and develop Alzheimer's?

I answer this question by telling female patients at my clinic: yes, if you improve your heart health, your risk of Alzheimer's and depression will decrease. Science has not yet answered this question with absolute certainty, but remember: it took fifty years for science to prove that smoking causes cancer, yet doctors working with lung cancer patients quickly made the connection. From my extensive work with patients suffering from all of these terrible diseases, I can say with certainty that heart health is brain health is body health.

We now know that heart disease risk is *different* for women and men, not that women are at *less* risk of heart disease. Yes, more men have heart disease, but with heart disease killing more women than any other ailment, the fact that the disease is more prevalent in men is hardly relevant to women's health. Without a doubt, medicine has been making mistakes in women's heart health for over a century.

To complicate matters, the American lifestyle today is a breeding ground for chronic disease. Throughout Part II, you will learn about the heart health ramifications of foods that are poison to optimal functioning, our exposure to hundreds of toxic chemicals (starting before birth), and living the most sedentary lives in human history. Although we live twice as long as our ancestors, a strong argument can be made that we are truly healthy for fewer years than our ancestors were.

Despite widely disseminated health information that makes us more aware than ever that our lifestyle will influence our future health, most people today continue to lead lives and eat foods that greatly increase their risk of chronic disease and decrease the quality of their lives. I can say with complete conviction that, for optimal health, most of the foods available in the grocery store should not be consumed and we should not spend half our lives sitting at desks, in cars, and on sofas.

There are encouraging trends in health, however, and lifestyle options that support heart health are more accessible than they've ever been. We can buy organic foods at big-box megastores, and supply and demand have lowered the price of high-quality natural foods. The new media of the information age have warned millions of people about the dangers of consuming sugary drinks, processed carbohydrates, and trans fats. Outdoor sports and a variety of gym-based activities have become more diverse, easier and safer to do, and available to more people than ever before. Heart-healthy lifestyle trends like yoga and rock climbing are skyrocketing in popularity and now appeal to people who may have traditionally eschewed activities of this kind.

If you're reading this book, you're already one of the people moving our culture of health in the right direction. Yet, despite the efforts of women like you who care deeply about their health and other efforts to improve women's heart health knowledge, both scientifically and culturally, women's heart health is still suffering a hangover from years of neglect.

The ponderous battleship of modern medicine is slow to turn. Until lifestyle and nutrition medicine is practiced on an individual basis—doctors working with each patient to develop personalized recommendations rather than simply giving all patients mainstream medicine's generic recommendations or prescriptions for dangerous pills—it is up to people like you to take the initiative and treat your heart with the care it deserves. You can do that by taking advantage of the pleasurable and diverse opportunities available today to improve your heart health, completing the self-assessment found in the following pages, and adapting the life-enhancing methods provided here to your unique lifestyle and physiology.

Heart health is inseparably tied to a vast array of ailments, ranging from acute heart issues like heart attack and stroke to the more chronic conditions of diabetes, high blood pressure, obesity, chronic fatigue, fibromyalgia, irritable bowel, and, as mentioned earlier, even brain conditions such as Alzheimer's, and depression. There is both good news and bad news from these emerging relationships between heart health and not only heart disease but other chronic ailments. The bad news—as you might already have guessed—is that, if we've been neglecting women's heart health, then we must admit that we've also been neglecting women's overall health and leaving them at higher risk of this plethora of other chronic diseases. The good news is that personalized lifestyle medicine has given us the tools to drastically reduce not only heart disease risk but also the other symptoms and diseases associated with heart health. Additionally, thanks to the efforts of my esteemed peers and organizations like the Personalized Lifestyle Medicine Institute and the Institute for Functional Medicine, we now have proof that these methods actually work.

Following the lead of the inspiring strides already made against chronic disease—such as Dr. Dean Ornish's heart disease reversal program, Dr. Amy Myers's autoimmune plan, Dr. Aviva Romm's adrenal thyroid revolution, Dr. Sara Gottfried's age resistance program, functional medicine practitioner Marcelle Pick's hormone balance program, and Dr. Mark Hyman's blood sugar therapies—my goal in *Heart Solution for Women* is to apply the principles of functional medicine to women's specific physiology and present the lifestyle therapies and solutions used by physicians in a way that will allow you, the reader, to reap many of the rewards of functional medicine, even without a visit to a functional medicine physician. This book will shatter the misconceptions about women's heart health, reveal pre–heart disease symptoms, and help women self-diagnose their own level of heart disease risk at any stage of life, and ultimately present a proven, personalized program to heal the heart.

The Case for Lifestyle Medicine

When a woman comes into my office to work with me on creating a plan to improve her health, she is the smartest person in the building. I help her trust her intuition and discuss her characteristics that indicate disease risk, but *she* is the one who decides where to focus her healing effort. This book is premised on the very same assumption—that you are in charge of your own health.

The majority of the recommendations presented here are not only effective at solving complex issues but also surprisingly simple to implement. We begin by looking at the factors that detract from optimal health. Then I'll help you evaluate your own imbalances and weak points where disease might take hold. Finally, we'll work together to design a custom program to strengthen and balance your health based on your specific issues. This is exactly what I do in my clinic. In this book, I will share those parts of the lifestyle medicine I practice that are safe to experiment with and can largely be self-directed without physician oversight. These "heart solutions" are not just theoretical or ideological, but elements of cutting-edge therapies that are proving more effective than drugs or surgeries in preventing and reversing chronic heart disease.

There's more good news. Lifestyle medicine has the pleasant side effect of making life better.

As my patients can confirm, these therapies to improve heart health will make you feel stronger, happier, leaner, sexier, more energetic, and otherwise more vital and resilient. The great thing about solutions to achieve optimal heart health is that many of them involve activities that enhance the quality of life. How nice would it be to walk out of a doctor's office with a prescription for learning, dancing, music, play, good food, and socializing? That's the kind of prescription I write for my patients—and what I hope to give you in this book.

The coming pages are filled with the latest on life-changing methodology from the front lines of functional medicine, but before we start, we need to get past a few common misconceptions. Many of you probably think of heart disease as a problem only for old or overweight individuals. So long as you're young, or thin, or watch your cholesterol intake (or take cholesterol drugs), or all of the above, you don't have anything to worry about, right? Hardly. It turns out that heart health and the diseases associated with it—everything from dementia to diabetes— don't fit into simple sound bites or blanket recommendations.

Diabetes is one of the flock of canaries in the coal mine of heart disease. Data from the vast amount of research that has been conducted on this ailment clearly show that the fight against diabetes may have reduced its occurrence in men, but is not helping women. Between 1971 and 2000, death rates for men with diabetes decreased by nearly 20 people per 1,000—yet there was no change in the death rate for women over the same period. Even so, the American Diabetes Association engages in the age-old practice of misrepresenting heart disease risk in women by comparing it to men's risk. Its 2018 website reads:

> Whether you're male or female also affects how likely you are
> to develop heart disease. Men are more likely to develop heart
> disease. But once a woman reaches menopause, her risk for

heart disease goes up. But even then, women still aren't as likely as men.

Heart disease is the number-one killer of women—*isn't that likely enough?* The problem is that the statistics used by those who make such statements tell only part of the story. Yes, more men than women suffer from diabetes (and heart disease), but when women do become diabetic (or have a stroke or heart attack), they usually fare worse than men. In addition, women are being left behind as the diabetes rates in men go down, and women's diabetes rates remain the same year after year. According to the results of the iconic Framingham Heart Study—one of the earliest heart disease studies to include women and still one of the most referenced and respected heart and lifestyle studies—the prevalence of heart failure in men and women is the same between the ages of fifty and fifty-nine, greater in women between the ages of eighty and eighty-nine, and about the same in men and women overall between the ages of twenty-five and seventy-four.

Another example of women drawing the short straw when it comes to heart disease is stroke, the fourth-leading cause of death in women. During the decade after menopause, the risk of stroke doubles in women, and although men have a higher risk of stroke than women at younger ages, women make up 60 percent of stroke victims. Many studies have shown that after suffering a stroke, women tend to fare worse than men: they leave the hospital in worse condition, recover more slowly, and are more limited in their activities for a longer period of time.

The Heart of a Woman

It is clear that the medical profession has a lot of work to do to change its approach to women's heart health, but the cultural side of this issue also presents enormous challenges. If even most doctors haven't been given women-specific heart information and don't really understand women's heart health, how are everyday people supposed to understand it? For instance, only half of the female population knows that heart disease is the number-one killer of women. To raise awareness, Barbra Streisand helped launch the Women's Heart Alliance and a Fight the Ladykiller educational campaign. Even with strong voices like Streisand's trying to tell the truth about heart disease, most of the women I talk to in my clinic are more worried about breast cancer— even though they are five times more likely to die of heart disease.

Complicating matters are the physical differences between men's and women's hearts and vascular systems, which contribute in surprising ways to the misunderstandings about women's heart health. While the average man stands only about five inches taller than the average woman, women's hearts are fully 20 *percent* smaller *than men's hearts*—a greater proportional difference than their difference in height. This difference in the heart sizes of men and women isn't entirely understood; one *American Heart Association* journal article concluded that "neither body size nor clinical status can fully compensate for the discrepancies in heart size between the sexes." The difference in heart size relative to body size means that, to pump the same amount of blood, a woman's heart has to beat more rapidly than the 20 percent larger heart of a man of the same body size. Thus, the average woman's resting heart ticks along about 10 beats per minute faster than the average man's.

It would seem that this difference in size should be easy to adjust for in determining something as important as heart health, but it's not so simple. Electrocardiograms (ECGs), the classic heart monitor used in every hospital and emergency room—as well as in every Hollywood emergency room movie and television scene—are not as accurate on women. This inaccuracy too often results, surprisingly, in a false negative: the device indicates that a woman is not having a heart attack when, in fact, she is.

The most common dysfunction of the heart valves, mitral valve disease, is equally common in both men and women, but for men the incidence is the same across all age groups, while for women it occurs most often in younger women. Also, the deadly plaque that forms on the walls of arteries, causing heart attacks, collects differently in men than in women: in men, plaque collects in clumps that are easily seen in an angiogram (an X-ray of blood flow), while the plaque in women's arteries tends to be more evenly collected throughout and harder to see, making an accurate risk assessment more difficult.

The carotid artery, which runs up the neck and supplies the brain's voracious appetite for oxygen and nutrients, is the second-biggest artery in the body. To reduce the risk for stroke, a procedure called a carotid endarterectomy (CEA) can be performed to remove material that has built up in the artery. In a seeming contradiction, a woman who has material built up in her carotid artery, even though it is smaller than a man's carotid artery, is at lower risk of a blockage in that artery causing stroke. How a smaller artery can result in a lower risk of stroke is baffling, but such are the mysteries of the human body, and the unexpected differences between women's and men's hearts and vascular systems. Compounding the issue, complication rates for CEAs performed on women are higher than for men, causing some researchers to suggest that for women the benefits of undergoing this invasive procedure do not outweigh the risks.

These are not insignificant differences. In 2015, a Johns Hopkins School of Medicine study determined that, in women, the heart muscle that encircles the main chamber of the heart either gets smaller or stays the same size as they age. In men, however, this muscle grows larger and thicker. Dr. João Lima, the senior author of the study, said, "Our results are a striking demonstration that heart disease may have a different pathophysiology in men and women, and of the need for tailored treatments that address such important biologic differences."

After reading these last few pages, do you feel like you have less risk of heart disease than the men you know? Do you think your doctor has been given the right information to help you protect your heart? Have you concluded that you don't have to worry about heart disease because you're a woman? Just writing these pages made me think about my daughter and how her heart is so different from mine. What a disservice it is to her to summarize her heart health by simply saying she has less risk of heart disease than I do as a man. For my daughter, my mother, my patients, and you as my reader, I find it utterly absurd to evaluate your heart disease risk only relative to men. I want to help you lower your personal risk, period—not your heart disease risk compared to other people's, and least of all your risk compared to men's.

Caring for your heart is how you reduce your own personal risk, and that's what I'm going to show you how to do. If I could choose the one message you'll remember after learning about the problem in Part I, discovering how your heart interacts with the rest of your body in Part II, and building your own precise and personalized heart health solution in Part III, it would be that you have every right to demand— from both yourself and your doctor—the highest-quality heart care.

The Illusion of the Easy Solution

Making matters even worse for women's heart health, our issues in treating chronic disease go far beyond gender. Perhaps most significantly, modern medicine and our culture are deeply permeated by the illusion that drugs, surgeries, and intensive care will save us from chronic problems. These methods work incredibly well for those suffering from a problem with a clear and singular cause, like a bacterial infection or a traumatic injury. With chronic diseases that develop over a long period of time, however, relying on drugs or surgeries far too often is counterproductive. Because pharmaceuticals work so well for acute ailments, too many of us assume that they also work—or that an effective medication will soon be invented—to cure chronic disease. This assumption has the dangerous effect of enabling people to rationalize health-damaging behavior because they feel a drug will take care of them. The unfortunate reality is that, despite decades of research in the best and most capable drug laboratories on the planet, drugs are proving to be a poor solution to chronic disease.

The gold standard of medical progress, the clinical trial, has been extremely beneficial to medicine; however, the clinical trial is also deeply flawed when it comes to solving an individual's health problems— particularly when multiple body systems, symptoms, and causes are involved. The ideal clinical trial has every element under absolute control and requires a control group—a group of people who are not undergoing the therapy. To create a clinical trial that could provide absolute scientific evidence that a particular heart health therapy is right for you, we would need to find hundreds of people with very similar symptoms, food sensitivities, diet, lifestyle, medical history, and even genetics. We would then have to give half of them the optimal treatment while subjecting the control group to daily stress, poor diet, toxin exposure, and little or no exercise, love, or support. Not only would this clinical trial be impossible, it would also be unethical.

Another issue is that much of the research into medications based on clinical trials is funded by drug companies. Although the pharmaceutical industry is responsible for some of the greatest leaps in medicine, scientific research conducted by the industry on its own products—research that drives medical protocol—is inevitably fraught with issues. To put it simply, industry-funded studies are designed to have a desired result, and when that result is not forthcoming, some studies may not even make it to publication.

Then there is the issue that we don't like to talk about: unhealthy lifestyles are incredibly good for the economy. Fast food alone generates $200 billion annually in the United States, and that figure doesn't include revenues from sales of the equally damaging cereals, sodas, and processed foods that line grocery store aisles. Add alcohol, cigarettes, and sedentary entertainment to the equation and it's no stretch to say that the bad-for-us industry is an enormous part of the global economy.

On the other side of the economic machine of ill health, Big Pharma makes billions of dollars off of our modern pill-for-the-ill culture. The pharmaceutical industry is consistently at the top of the list of the most profitable industries. In 2016, generic pharmaceuticals topped that list with a 30 percent profit margin; the automobile industry, for comparison, had about a 5 percent margin.

Then there's the natural foods and health industry, which also taps into the wallets of people who don't feel as good as they should. Supplements are all the rage, with every natural food store and pharmacy lined with aisle after aisle of tinctures, tablets, oils, and salves claiming to help solve all kinds of issues. I'm a huge fan of supplements—used in a way that targets an individual's unique vitamin and nutrient deficits, they form a key part of the "Precision, Personalized Solution" presented in Part III—but not all supplements are created equal and not every person will respond the same way to a particular supplement. I even started my own line of high-quality nutritional supplements and protein smoothies to ensure that I could recommend products that I am absolutely sure will help my patients. The quality of the active ingredients in supplements varies dramatically: some are made in cutting-edge laboratories with exacting standards, and others in outdoor labs with no quality control whatsoever. The inactive ingredients in supplements are at least as much of an issue: the binders and fillers in some supplements prevent absorption even when the nutrient or vitamin in the supplement is high-quality. I'll have more to say about this in Chapter 8.

The alternative health industry has tapped into the health dollars pipeline as well, promising all sorts of benefits while presenting little or no evidence that many of these claims actually work. There is vast potential in alternatives to mainstream medicine—in fact, using alternative medicine in combination with mainstream medicine is what I do. But the alternative health industry has done itself no favors by selling billions of dollars' worth of products that claim to improve health but often do nothing and sometimes even make matters worse. The Federal Food, Drug, and Cosmetic Act of 1938 made it illegal to market and sell products that claim to prevent, diagnose, treat, mitigate, or cure diseases without demonstrating that the products are safe and effective for their labeled uses, but there are many ways in which companies get around this law. Since 1994, the US Food and Drug Administration (FDA) has identified 300 products that either do not do what they claim or contain ingredients not permitted in dietary products. We're not talking about just truth in advertising either: people have suffered strokes, kidney and liver failure, and heart palpitations after consuming these products, and some have even died.

It's a vicious circle, but sick people are good for business. I'm part of the health industry too. Pharmaceuticals, vitamins, and supplements have been some of the greatest boons to humankind, and I prescribe them daily in my practice. Due in part to my master's degree trainings in pharmacology, I ask all new patients to bring their drugs, supplements, and vitamins to the first appointment. In my opinion, after seeing the incredible collections of pills that most of them bring into my office, I can say with certainty that the vast majority of prescriptions, supplements, and over-the-counter medicines being taken are not helping. Supplements or medications that don't get to the heart of the problem may, at best, either mask symptoms or do nothing; at worst, they add to the problem.

Finally, our spend-it-now-pay-for-it-later lifestyle sets a terrible trap for many people. We all know that defaulting on financial debt can result in poor credit. But we can just declare bankruptcy and erase our debts, right? Well, there is no bankruptcy court for health. Eating poorly, living a stressed-out life, and then looking for cures after getting sick is a poor business model, yet many feel stuck in it. If you're following a fast-food, high-stress lifestyle, you will almost certainly pay the price for excess sugar, inadequate nutrition, systemic inflammation, and stress response—and then receive medical intervention *after* the symptoms of disease appear. It's a bit like trying to solve the problem of an overflowing sink by mopping up the water spilling over the sides rather than turning off the faucet.

Until our culture and the way we practice medicine change significantly, a healthy person who wants to preserve her function, or a person who is beginning to suffer chronic issues and wants to heal before it's too late, will be best served by considering her unique symptoms, family history, aerobic condition, and food sensitivities—and then changing her lifestyle accordingly. After using these strategies to evaluate and help thousands of patients, I realized that everyone can do most of what my patients do to heal without even going to the doctor. These treatments are not expensive. They're not dangerous. And they make life better.

This why I wrote this book; to show you how to heal yourself using much of what I do as a functional medicine physician.

But before we get into the action plan, the first step on the path to improved health is learning how to balance systems far from the heart. For your heart cannot be truly healthy if the rest of your body is a hotbed of inflammation, off-kilter from the side effects of powerful medications, functioning with a natural detoxification system overloaded with environmental toxins, and thrown far out of balance by the hormones and internal messaging blown around like leaves in the wind by your genetic and lifestyle factors.

In Chapter 2, you'll learn about the pervasive myths of heart disease and finally discover the truth about cholesterol, statins, surgery, diets, and more. In Chapter 3, I'll show you why inflammation is at the heart of heart disease and help you find the little things you're doing all day long that spark an inflammatory response. In Chapters 4 and 5, you'll learn all about what I call the "functional medicine quartet"—the four systems in your body that work together to keep you healthy—and you'll discover how food, toxins, bugs, and trauma mess with your hormones and therefore with your heart.

Part III is where you'll assess your own risk factors and create your Precision, Personalized Solution. Chapters 6 through 9 provide you with a guide to food, exercise, and supplements as well as a highly individualized program that you can take with you for the rest of your life. Throughout the book, you'll learn how your specific body type is contributing to disease and the individual healing strategies that will work best for you—the very same process we would go through if you came into my clinic as a patient.

The Deception of Diagnosis

Amy was forty-four years old when she first visited my clinic, having already been diagnosed with several serious diseases to account for her extremely poor quality of life: chronic fatigue at age thirty-two, fibromyalgia at thirty-three, and multiple sclerosis at forty-one. Her symptoms included widespread pain, muscle weakness, deep depression, anxiety, and panic attacks, poor sleep without recovery upon waking, and debilitating fatigue. She had seen multiple doctors and was on—and addicted to—several strong medications. Amy's husband estimated that she had only about 10 percent function, with only enough energy to go to the bathroom and then back to bed.

It's been three years since Amy visited my clinic. The therapies that helped her are the same ones found in this book—a combination of lifestyle medicine, and the body's incredible ability to heal. By correcting a few imbalances rather than treating single severe symptoms, I was able to help Amy regain her body's balance and change her life in dramatic and lasting ways.

I helped Amy find a solution by looking beyond her most painful symptoms and showing her tools she could use in her daily life to regain internal balance. I did prescribe low doses of safe pharmaceuticals that would have minimal side effects, but the majority of the therapies that helped balance her systems involved changing her food choices and taking a couple of targeted high-quality supplements. Amy continues to follow the protocol we designed together, and she steadily continues to improve to this day. After receiving truly horrendous diagnoses that left her feeling she would never have the energy for the grocery store, much less for school, work, family, and life, Amy will have finished beauty school and will be enjoying her new career by the time you read this.

Amy's issues were not easily categorized as certain diseases. She was suffering serious health conditions, but medicine's definition of "disease" did not adequately describe her overall health condition. Most importantly, Amy's solution lay in addressing the underlying condition, not in treating her symptoms.

I hope you are not suffering from nearly as dire a situation as Amy's, but you almost certainly have internal systems that are out of balance, reducing your function and increasing your heart disease risk and maybe even setting you up for a future heart disease diagnosis. By seeking harmony between your bodily systems and taking steps toward improved vitality by applying the program in this book to your life like Amy did to hers, you will improve your quality of life and reduce your risk of disease, heart and otherwise.

With all this in mind, it should be obvious that, rather than waiting for menopause or an actual disease diagnosis before thinking about your heart health and beginning a program of healing, it is far better to start pursuing heart-healing lifestyle medicine as soon as possible. This approach—building resistance to disease and healing deeply hidden wounds—forms the basis of functional medicine, whose goal is to improve people's lives by emphasizing their unique story, intuition, medical history, and desire to heal as much as their test results, the bell curve of averages and published conclusions. Practitioners of functional medicine value the evidence provided by clinical studies, but we also consider the individual's improvement as the most valuable evidence of all. This focus on the individual is at the heart, so to speak, of the Heart Solution for Women.

One critical aspect of finding your personal solution is a mind shift—a change in your thinking about disease. Disease is not a stark line we cross from a state of health into a state of illness. Rather, we all have the seeds of disease already lurking and growing within us. The classic risk factors for heart disease include obesity, high cholesterol levels, smoking, high blood pressure, family history, age, poor diet, and stress. Diabetes, a condition that involves excess blood sugar, is also considered a risk factor for heart disease, but the argument could be made that diabetes *is* heart disease. Blood sugar balance is a condition that has been identified as a concern worthy of consideration, and intervention, not only after crossing that imaginary line into disease but long before a disease diagnosis. If, in diabetes, we designate the state of increasing blood sugar as "pre-diabetic," doesn't it make sense to think of the other risk factors for heart disease as "pre–heart disease"? Shouldn't we consider any path leading toward disease worthy of diagnosis and treatment? If it were up to me, pre-stress, pre-obesity, pre–high blood pressure, and pre–high cholesterol would be just as carefully considered and researched as the diseases implicated by these risk factors.

Own It

Since medicine is only just beginning to tap into the healing potential of individualized lifestyle medicine, the best way for you to find your unique seeds of disease and prevent them from growing is with a program designed by you, optimized for you, and managed by you. Lifestyle medicine programs have proven effective at healing individuals whose bodies have been damaged by stroke, heart attack, or the other debilitating and deadly conditions related to heart health. The Heart Solution for Women and other similar programs are at the cutting edge of chronic disease medicine.

Your individual solution may include blood tests or, depending on your fitness level, oversight from a personal trainer to find your optimal exercise level. But most of the therapies explained in this book can be applied inexpensively, safely, and with vitality-enhancing results in your own home, at work, and at the store, and with no collaboration other than the support of your partner or loved ones. Even in a case as severe as Amy's, 90 percent of the therapies involved ingredients available without prescriptions or physician oversight. Amy explained her solution best when she said: "Dr. Mark saved my life. No, Dr. Mark showed me how to save my own."

Amy's perspective sums up the only reliable way I've found to help people prevent, reverse, and heal from heart disease and other chronic diseases: *Show them how to do it themselves.*

Before we move on to Chapter 2, let's revisit Sue. In the beginning of this chapter, you learned that, after her near-miss with gallbladder surgery, Sue went in for a heart assessment. Her cardiologist determined that she had a severely damaged heart muscle. She would not regain function, he told her, and was facing a drastically limited future as a cardiac cripple.

But that future was not to be. Our emerging understanding of the heart suggests that damaged heart muscle is best described as hibernating, not dead, and that it can often be revived through targeted nutritional intervention, including coenzyme Q^{10}, carnitine, magnesium, and D-ribose. All of these supplements, which you'll learn about in Part III, are available over the counter at many health food stores.

For Sue's recovery plan, we put her on a personalized heart restoration nutrient protocol and a custom exercise program of activities that anyone could do on their own. Six months later, she met her cardiologist at a half-marathon. Yes, she was running—and she was anything but a cardiac cripple.

The beautiful part of Sue's story is that even though she was misdiagnosed, treated for her heart attack three days too late, and given a horrible prognosis, she went on to run a half-marathon less than a year after her heart attack. For both Amy and Sue, can you imagine what the incredible healing power of their own bodies could have achieved had they begun using the simple and effective strategies I'm providing in these pages years, or even decades, earlier?

Changing your lifestyle is daunting. The patients I've had who were best able to meet this challenge were those in charge of their own solution—not because I told them what to do, and not because the science clearly shows that lifestyle choices can either cause or prevent disease. They succeeded in changing their lifestyle because they made the process theirs and theirs alone.

Any woman can use the Heart Solution for Women, but it is how you as an individual customize this program and bring together its separate elements that will make it a useful, effective, achievable solution for you. This is why it is important to make lifestyle medicine part of who you are as soon as possible. The results will not be the same if you start this program ten years from now. As we age, the damaging factors of our lifestyle and our genetics become more difficult to modify and harder to heal, so the sooner you initiate your solution, the better it will work. Every one of my patients can vouch for this: life is better with a healthier heart. When you create a lifestyle medicine program perfectly tailored to yourself, and then follow it long enough, it will become not lifestyle medicine, but quite simply life itself.

Chapter 2

Cholesterol, Statins, Surgery, and Other Myths About Heart Disease

After reading Chapter 1, you may be feeling irritated, even angry, that you and millions of other women have been misled and overlooked. I hate to say it, but I'm glad you feel this way. Irritation and anger are powerfully motivating emotions that I can help you harness and channel into a knowledge- and empowerment-based program to improve your life along with your heart. Unfortunately, in addition to the sad state of women's heart care, the story of heart disease doesn't end with the imbalance of heart care between the genders. The pervasive myths about heart disease involving cholesterol, fat, statins, surgery, and more, which keep both women and men from finding a solution in the halls of conventional medicine, demonstrate why we need to entirely rethink how we treat this terrible disease.

From how much cholesterol to consume to a misguided focus on "dieting" and vastly overused and dangerous statin drug prescriptions, my patients often arrive at my clinic terribly confused about what their tests mean, what to eat, and what pills, prescriptions, or treatments to pursue. I want to put an end to all of the confusion right now.

If you are reading this book and have concerns about your heart health, chances are you know a little bit about heart disease and the systems at work in your body. You've probably heard of "good" and "bad" cholesterol and been told that you need to monitor your intake of cholesterol in general. You may also know that the manipulation of cholesterol is controversial and that some fats are dangerous and others are healthy. We're about to dive deep into the myths of cholesterol and other misunderstandings around heart disease, but first we have to take a step back and answer a simple question: *What is heart disease?*

In your lifetime, your heart will fill and empty at least 2.5 billion times. It beats about 100,000 times daily and over 40 million times yearly. It will pump over a million barrels of blood, and even when you are sitting quietly, it will do twice as much work as your leg muscles in an all-out sprint. Every hour your heart pumps about 100 gallons of blood through a vascular system consisting of 60,000 miles of blood vessels. If lined up end to end, these vessels would wrap around the world at the equator—twice. It follows that the layer of cells lining your blood vessels, the endothelium, is the largest organ in your body. (The next time someone tells you the largest organ is the skin, you can set them straight.)

The vast majority of us are born with perfect hearts and optimally functioning vascular systems, but over time, and through a wide range of insults, our hearts, veins, arteries, and the rest of the nutrient delivery systems that nurture our hearts suffer damage that can eventually cause disease—and all too often does. From where I sit, working every day to help people heal their hearts, the definition of heart disease is a line in the sand, not an absolute definition or condition. Fundamentally, heart disease is anything that damages the heart. If you Google "heart disease," you'll get a range of heart-related diseases and definitions, even among high-quality peer-reviewed sources. It's not that these definitions are wrong. It's just a matter of where the authors are focused—where they draw the line.

To understand heart disease, let's start with the end point of the disease and work backwards from there. In medical school, I was taught that heart disease happens when your artery slowly fills up with cholesterol plaque until there is only one little opening left. Then, when you have your next super-size burger at the nearest fast-food joint, that little opening is plugged with fatty food, the artery stops the blood flow, and boom!—you're having a heart attack. Then we were taught that taking an aspirin somehow magically protects you from this process. As it turns out, this is not what happens at all.

The problem is caused not so much by large plaques plugging the artery, but rather by a plaque of any size becoming inflamed or irritable and rupturing. Think of an inflamed plaque as being like a zit in your heart artery. It may be big or small and may start as a little red spot that develops into a puss-filled whitehead and pops. This rupture alerts the body's strong defense system to deploy to fix a wound and your blood cells, called platelets, rush in to fix that little hole. The inflammation caused by the wound makes the platelets sticky, so they clump together. If the inflammation causes the platelets to overreact to the small hole, they create a clot large enough to block the entire artery, and if the artery isn't flexible enough to accommodate the clot, you have a heart attack. Once the heart muscle loses its oxygen flow, it begins to die within minutes—and so do you.

This is *coronary artery disease,* and it's what most people think of when they talk about heart disease. Its most common conclusion is heart attack, accounting for about half of all heart disease victims. And here's the scary part: in one half of women who suffer plaque rupture in the heart artery that causes a blockage, the first warning sign is sudden death. Many women don't get a second chance when it comes to heart disease.

Another end point of heart disease is stroke, which is what happens when arterial blockage due to a blood clot occurs in one of the blood vessels that supply blood to the brain. Because it's the brain being affected, not the heart, some lists of heart diseases don't include stroke, but the conditions that cause stroke are exactly the same as those that cause a heart attack. (And on the bright side, the lifestyle medicine that prevents heart attack also prevents stroke.) Stroke accounts for another one-third of heart disease victims.

Other far less prevalent forms of heart disease include birth defects (exceedingly rare), heart valve disease, which prevents the heart valves from opening enough to let adequate blood pass, and heart rhythm dysfunction, which is the heart beating too fast, too slow, or out of rhythm. These conditions make up a small fraction of heart disease cases and are not as closely related to lifestyle as stroke and coronary artery disease. Thus, these conditions are not the primary focus of the *Heart Solution for Women*. That said, the program described here will improve virtually every system in the body in beautiful ways, so the optimization of the heart that accompanies adherence to an effective lifestyle medicine program may prevent other heart-specific diseases, as well as other diseases not even mentioned in this book, from fully developing.

Our focus here, however, is to improve heart function in tangible and dramatic ways in order to prevent the final, deadly, acute manifestations of heart disease: heart attack and stroke. With this goal in mind, several other heart-related diseases enter the game: high blood pressure, obesity, hypercholesterolemia (extremely high cholesterol), and type 2 diabetes. These diseases do not develop in isolation within the heart, but because they can ultimately kill a person through heart attack or stroke, many doctors and scientists consider them to be heart disease.

The list of causes of heart disease doesn't stop there. One of the pillars of functional medicine is the study of how inflammation originating in one part of the body affects the function of the rest of the body's systems. This isn't just a theory. There are now troves of evidence showing that inflammation is a primary driver of many kinds of disease, including heart disease. Thus, the way each individual's inflammatory defense reacts to food, bugs, trauma, toxins, and other stress becomes a significant factor in the development of heart disease.

Dysfunction of the arteries or the heart itself is heart disease. Obesity is heart disease. Diabetes is heart disease. High blood pressure is heart disease. Extremely high or low cholesterol is heart disease. And I'd even take it a step further and say that runaway inflammation is heart disease. It's a scary laundry list, but remember: all of these conditions can be manipulated by the individual with the tools presented in this book and readily available just about anywhere in the modern world. Now, with these defining factors of heart disease in mind, let's clear up a mountain of myths that have developed around the disease.

The following is a summary of what I consider the top seven myths about heart disease—and the realities, based on the latest peer-reviewed research and my own work healing thousands of patients, that debunk them. This chapter will not only enlighten you on the pervasive myths of heart disease but teach you about what really drives disease development, why our current trend of consuming low-cholesterol and low-fat foods is flawed, why statin drugs hurt more people than they help, and more. Once you understand these myths, you'll have a more clear perspective from which to consider the lessons of Part II, where I'll help you learn how the systems of your body can either become susceptible to disease or resist and heal from disease.

MYTH #1: High cholesterol levels cause heart disease

➤ **The reality:** Half the people who suffer heart attacks have normal cholesterol levels

In the early years of the research into what causes heart disease, the cholesterol connection was a logical concept to pursue. In the 1700s, the cardiologist Friedrich Hoffmann made the connection between heart disease and reduced blood flow in the coronary arteries. Early autopsies of heart attack victims revealed that the material obstructing their arteries resembled common foods such as butter, lard, or beef tallow, so researchers concluded that some kind of fat seemed to be the culprit. Improved technology eventually allowed scientists to see that these fatty obstructions contained fibrin, cholesterol, calcium, and other fatty materials. Seeming to confirm the visual evidence was the circumstantial evidence that heart attacks were more common in countries where people ate large amounts of fats.

In the early 1900s, a Russian researcher named Nikolay Anichkov found what many considered to be a smoking gun with cholesterol's fingerprints all over it. When rabbits were fed purified cholesterol for several months, their blood cholesterol levels rose dramatically, and autopsies showed fatty materials obstructing their hearts and arteries. Anichkov had discovered a link between cholesterol and damage to the heart far ahead of his time. However, because rabbits are vegetarians and do not eat fats or cholesterol, they don't have the omnivore or carnivore physiology to process fat. Also, the cholesterol-like matter causing the rabbits' arterial blockages had built up in a different manner from the obstructions that have been observed in human arteries. In the rabbits, the cholesterol was found to be adhering to the inner lining of the arterial walls; in humans, the cholesterol buildup is *within* the arterial walls.

Cholesterol is an essential element of the membranes of your body's cells, including those in the walls of your arteries. And the reality is that cholesterol is present around damaged arteries not because it *caused* the damage, but because the body uses it to *repair* damage.

The importance of cholesterol is underscored by the fact that every cell in your body has the capability to make it. Nutritional wisdom has put a lot of weight on dietary cholesterol, but only 10 percent of your cholesterol comes from your food—the other 90 percent is manufactured in your body, mostly in your liver. If you reduce your cholesterol levels too far, your body will make more. It is also an important molecule in your body's hormonal messaging, such as functions involving estrogen, testosterone, corticosteroids, and progesterone. Mother's milk is over 50 percent cholesterol.

Cholesterol's physiological benefits include:

- Increased libido (cholesterol-lowering statin drugs are associated with reduced sex drive)

- Helping your body eliminate toxins

- Helping build strong bones (and helping your body manufacture vitamin D, which is not a vitamin but a steroid hormone that is also important for the brain and immune system)

- Reducing the risk of cancer

- Supporting brain function

On that last benefit, you could say that we are all fat heads: 25 percent of the body's cholesterol is in the brain, and low cholesterol is associated with poor memory and reduced critical thinking. In fact, people over age sixty-five with the lowest cholesterol levels have the highest rates of dementia and memory problems.

So how do we square these benefits of cholesterol with the myth of high cholesterol? It's true that extremely high cholesterol can cause problems. But it's also true that a dangerously high cholesterol level is more often a symptom of dysfunction than a cause itself. For thirty years the medical community has been treating cholesterol as public enemy number one when in fact cholesterol is largely an innocent bystander who has taken the heat while the real criminals—inflammation, epigenetic response, high blood sugar and stress, to name a few—got away with murder. Literally.

The data just don't support high cholesterol as the driving factor in heart disease risk. Half of the people who suffer heart attacks have normal cholesterol levels and half have high cholesterol. The Framingham Heart Study, which has been following a group of individuals' cardiovascular health since 1948, revealed that *80 percent of all the individuals who had experienced a heart event had cholesterol levels similar to those of individuals who had not.*

MYTH #2: The total cholesterol test gives me a good measurement of my heart disease risk because it accurately measures my LDL and HDL cholesterol

> ➤ **The reality:** A standard cholesterol test score is a poor method for assessing heart disease risk because, by simply combining measurements of the bad LDL, the good HDL, and the inflammatory triglycerides and other small particles, it ignores the types of particle that make up bad LDL and good HDL cholesterol, which are what matter

As you now know, cholesterol plays a complicated biochemical role in your body that leaves a lot of room for manipulation of the facts. The cholesterol screening you'll receive from your average health insurer, for instance, is based on a calculation that grossly oversimplifies the way cholesterol works. These tests are only about 40 percent predictive of heart attack risk. The direct measurement cholesterol test (see Chapter 9), which breaks cholesterol down into more than twelve direct measurements and over fifteen inflammatory markers, may be over 95 percent predictive of heart attack risk. If I were your doctor, you would already have taken a direct measurement cholesterol test.

The idea of "good" and "bad" cholesterol wouldn't be nearly as confusing if we hadn't been told for decades that all cholesterol was bad. The way I like to explain it to my patients is that the good cholesterol, HDL, is a protective type of "carrier" cholesterol that helps to keep the bad LDL cholesterol in check. LDL has four subtypes, which tend to be either big fluffy, bouncy balls of LDL that are not so bad and don't tend to stick together, or small, dense, sticky LDL that tends to make dangerous, unstable plaques. The sticky stuff is the small dense LDL (sdLDL) and the lipoprotein (a) or Lp(a). Emerging research suggests that for women Lp(a) may be the most dangerous.

Making the LDL situation even worse is a particularly nasty kind of LDL called oxidized LDL (OxLDL). This "rusty cholesterol" builds up when the cholesterol interacts with free radicals in the body and becomes oxidized, increasing the amount of fat deposited in the body. This interaction in turn increases the oxidation of the LDL because oxidation and the release of free radicals are side effects of the body burning (metabolizing) the fat. It's an ugly, inflammatory cycle. Illustrating the complexity of cholesterol's role in the body is the fact that the best way to reduce OxLDL is to increase your HDL cholesterol, which literally sucks the OxLDL out of the arterial wall. This process is bolstered when you increase your antioxidant functions through nutrition, exercise, and perhaps supplements, which we'll talk about more in Part III.

I know—it's complicated. Let's look at two scenarios that may make it easier to understand the role of cholesterol in our bodies.

Jenny and Beth have the exact same high total cholesterol score and also the same high LDL "bad" score on the traditional calculated test. But Jenny has low levels of Lp(a). Her "bad" cholesterol isn't even all that bad; some of her LDL is the big, fluffy kind that has protective qualities for the heart. She eats a healthy, low-fat, high-vegetable diet and gets plenty of exercise. So Jenny actually has relatively low risk for a heart attack or stroke even though her total cholesterol and LDL score are both high.

Beth gets the same calculated LDL result as Jenny on the traditional cholesterol test, but Beth has high levels of Lp(a) and the small, sticky, dense sdLDL, and low levels of the big, fluffy, protective LDL. Beth's cholesterol also includes the "rusty" OxLDL, the most damaging kind of cholesterol. She eats a high-carb and sugar diet, with lots of industrially processed foods and factory-farmed, grain-fed red meat, and exercises only occasionally. Beth is at high risk for heart disease.

Based on their calculated cholesterol scores, both Jenny and Beth are prescribed statin drugs to lower their cholesterol. More about statins in a moment, but it's worth noting the likely outcomes. When the statin drugs lower her cholesterol, Beth, who actually does have dangerous cholesterol issues, doesn't change her lifestyle, since she figures the drugs will take care of her. But while her cholesterol numbers

Too Big to Fail

Three powerful forces aligned behind the bedeviling of cholesterol: the American Heart Association, pharmaceutical companies, and the food industry. For them, cholesterol was an ideal scapegoat and just happened to be oh so profitable.

The AHA recommended fat-free and low-fat products. The food industry partnered with the AHA and put AHA logos on its low-fat food products, which helped pay for AHA campaigns and was a powerful marketing tool for low-fat foods. The pharmaceutical companies sold billions of dollars of cholesterol-lowering statin drugs, among the most profitable pharmaceuticals in history. Through it all, everyone involved thought they were making healthy contributions to the war on heart disease.

Around the turn of the millennium, however, a better understanding of human biochemistry and biophysics began to emerge—an understanding that cleared cholesterol of many of its supposed crimes. As Dr. William Davis, author of the best-selling *Wheat Belly*, explains, "Today, you and I are able to directly quantify and characterize lipoproteins (fats), relegating

improve, the core imbalances that threaten her heart—inflammation, hormonal dysfunction, blood sugar levels—don't improve and in fact continue to worsen.

For Jenny, whose high levels of good cholesterol actually gave her added protection against heart disease, the statin drugs damage the mitochondria in her muscles and increase her insulin levels, both of which trigger cellular inflammation throughout her body. As a result, her blood pressure creeps higher. Jenny develops insulin sensitivity and eventually finds herself with diabetes and depression. Now she's in a high-risk category for heart disease—thanks to a drug that was supposed to lower her risk.

cholesterol to join the frontal lobotomies in the outdated medical garbage dump in the sky."

To put the accuracy of this comparison in perspective, the frontal lobotomy won a Nobel Prize in 1949—operating on the brains of the mentally ill was very much an accepted, common, and respected practice.

Unfortunately, by the time we figured out how cholesterol really works, the triad of forces aligned against it had grown too big to fail. No-fat and low-fat foods account for many billions of dollars of food product sales. Twenty-five million Americans are now on statin drugs with prescriptions for life, and the AHA can't just change its message overnight without losing credibility.

As it turns out, replacing dietary cholesterol and fat with carbohydrates and sugars (disguised to taste like fat in "fat-free" products) makes us fatter than eating fat in the first place! Even worse, replacing dietary cholesterol and fat with carbohydrates and sugars increases cellular inflammation, which increases the risk of heart disease.

Neither Jenny's doctor nor Beth's used a direct measurement cholesterol test, and neither was trained in individualized medicine; thus, neither Jenny nor Beth received the treatment they needed. If their doctors had been trained to look more deeply into the individual's specific fat types before prescribing statins, Beth and Jenny would have been given very different recommendations.

Beth may have needed the statin drug to address her high lipoprotein-a and sdLDL levels. At the same time, however, she also needed supplements to both protect her from the damaging effects of the statin and bolster her HDL good cholesterol, as well as a diet and exercise program tailored to her fitness level and perhaps an experimental period of using the powerful cholesterol-lowering supplement cocktail of niacin combined with high-quality red yeast rice extract (see Chapter 9) before committing to a lifetime prescription for statins. Taking these steps to improve her cholesterol scores might have spared her a lifetime prescription for statin drugs—and lowered her heart disease risk.

Jenny needed statin drugs like she needed a hole in the heart. If her doctor had taken a little more time with her to discuss the details of her diet, given her a direct measurement cholesterol test, and considered the big picture of her individual health, the doctor might have advised Jenny to increase her fish consumption, reduce her sugar and carbohydrate consumption, take a food sensitivity test, and switch from grain-fed to grass-fed beef (all part of the Heart Solution for Women). Rather than take a drug for life that may eventually cause diabetes and depression and therefore increase her heart disease risk, Jenny could have lowered her cholesterol in just a few months through lifestyle medicine and learning how to manage and improve her heart health without drugs.

MYTH #3: Fat is bad for the heart

➤ **The reality:** Eating more good fats and fewer bad fats will help to protect and heal your heart

One of the most controversial diet theories of all is that cholesterol and dietary fat should be avoided. This diet theory is also by far the most profitable, thanks to the popularity now of fat-replacement products sold as "low-fat" foods and the overprescribing of cholesterol-lowering drugs.

Listening to the experts and even reading the research on the subject do little to clear up the confusion around dietary fat. One of the most revealing studies on dietary fat and heart health in women was the Nurses' Health Study, which began in 1976 and involved over

120,000 female nurses between thirty and fifty-five years old. Each nurse completed a medical history and lifestyle questionnaire, and follow-up was conducted every two years through 1990.

Adjusting for age, the study showed that a significant increase in heart disease risk was associated with higher fat consumption. However, this connection disappeared when vigorous exercise, smoking, alcohol use, and vitamin E supplementation were taken into account. When these factors were considered in the analysis, the heart disease risk was found to be lowest among those who ate the least trans unsaturated fat (think margarine) and the most polyunsaturated fat (think fish oil). Eating more vegetable fat reduced the risk of developing heart disease, and increasing the amount of animal fat caused no change in risk at all. Researchers concluded that eating more saturated and trans fat increases the risk of heart disease, but that this risk is *decreased* by eating more monosaturated and polyunsaturated fats.

One of the most dramatic takeaways from the study, in my opinion, was what happened when the nurses *changed* the type of fat in their diet but did not reduce it. When they replaced just 2 percent of their calories from trans fat (such as red meat, shortening, and dairy) with those from unsaturated, unhydrogenated fat (from sources like fatty fish, nuts olive oil, and avocados), their risk of heart disease dropped by 53 percent. Clearly heart health is not as simple as just eating less fat.

To further complicate the picture, the experts differ dramatically in their recommendations. Dr. Dean Ornish recommends a low-fat diet with fat making up only 10 percent of total calories. Dr. Andrew Weil is a fan of a higher-fat diet with 30 percent of total calories coming from fat. Both are equally respected and well-studied, and both have shown success with their programs. In my experience, both are right, depending on the individual. What is right for you is different from what is right for the average person, especially since you don't want to be average—the new average in America is pre-diabetic and obese!

Fat is essential to heart health. It allows your body to process fat-soluble vitamins, helps with insulin response and blood sugar control, and sustains your energy levels (as opposed to the dreaded sugar crash). Fat supports hormone function, moderates mood swings, decreases brain fog, and reduces food cravings. We'll talk more about specific fats in Chapter 6, but for now it's important to know that healthy fat is an important part of heart-healing nutrition.

Numerous studies have come to the same conclusion about cholesterol and fats, and I'm hoping this book will convince you too that swapping "bad" fats for "good" fats favorably alters the lipid balance in your body. Your cells and system become more robust and function better, whereas reducing overall fat consumption in your diet would have little effect on your lipid balance or heart disease risk. Not only that, but replacing healthy fats with processed food advertised as "low-fat," as so many Americans have done, would almost certainly increase your heart disease risk.

If you're feeling a little confused about nutrition at this point, that's a good thing. Confusion is normal when we're throwing out old ideas in order to embrace new ones. The bottom line on dietary fat is this: unless you have extremely dangerous cholesterol levels, have already been diagnosed with coronary heart disease, or have suffered a stroke or heart attack, taking statin drugs or reducing your consumption of cholesterol and fats without considering the kind of fat you're consuming is likely to hurt you more than it helps you. (Stay tuned for my easy-to-remember guide to fats in Part III.)

MYTH #4: If I consume less cholesterol, I will be healthier

> ➤ **The reality:** If you consume less sugar, you will be healthier

With fat back on the table and cholesterol acquitted, let's talk about something we eat way too much of that is indeed causing heart disease: sugar.

Because sugar is not an essential nutrient, the FDA has not set an official recommended daily allowance (RDA) for it. Look at the nutrition label on the back of any food product containing sugar. You'll see the total sugar content measured in grams, but no RDA percentage.

There have been attempts to put an RDA on sugar, and the World Health Organization has recommended that no more than 10 percent of total calories come from sugar, but so far in America sugar remains a sacred cow.

Many suspect that the influence of the sugar lobby on government recommendations is responsible for the lack of an RDA. An even sneakier move is the sugar industry's funding of numerous studies that, while based on solid science, have shifted the media's focus away from sugar. Guess who funded the studies showing clearly that the more you sit the sooner you die? The sugar industry. Guess who funded many of the studies that show the benefits of dark chocolate? The sugar industry. Sure, sitting too much is bad, and some elements of dark chocolate are beneficial, but if you drink a soda at your stand-up desk or eat a Hershey's Special Dark chocolate bar that weighs 41 grams and contains 21 grams of sugar, you're almost certainly doing yourself more damage than if you'd kept your seat and eaten an apple. (Better still would be moving and changing positions frequently and eating the apple instead of the high-sugar chocolate bar.)

Thanks in part to studies like these, nearly unlimited sugar consumption is largely accepted as normal in the kitchens, lunch boxes, and school cafeterias of America. As shown in the documentary *Fed Up*, between 2008 and 2010 junk-food advertising targeted at children increased 60 percent, and 80 percent of public schools had deals with Coke or Pepsi to install sugar dispensers (soda vending machines). Even much of the so-called health food found in natural foods stores is sugar- and carbohydrate-based. As a result, many health food consumers suffer the same insults to their metabolism, insulin, and energy as people who eat junk food and drink soda. Americans spend $40 billion each year trying to lose weight, yet we consume an average of 150 pounds of sugar each year per person. What's more, almost one-third of that sugar is high-fructose corn syrup (HFCS)—one of the most fattening, inflammatory substances you can eat.

Many people think that excess weight can be eliminated by choosing different food products, ones that are branded as healthier. They choose "diet" soft drinks, "low-fat" ice cream, reduced-fat margarine, and "lite" beer. Recent research has taught us that aspartame, a sugar substitute commonly used in low-fat products, is a hormone disruptor and causes weight gain, not weight loss! Are you thinking about the products in your pantry and refrigerator right now? If so, bookmark this page, take a break from reading, and go toss any highly processed products labeled "low-fat" you have in the garbage.

Now that you have disposed of some of the more damaging foods in your house, consider this: because the diet versions of food products are less filling, we tend to eat and drink more of them. This tendency is a food industry dream come true, but the health consequences are enormous. In my observation, temporary diets and reduced-fat food products are more damaging to heart health than eating full-fat foods and never dieting for weight loss.

Are you looking at replacing your high-fat or high-sugar product with another product that promises the same taste and nutrition but with less sugar and fat? You'd be better off seeking out a food that satisfies the same nutritional need with less sugar and fat, not a "low-fat" or "sugar-free" version of the same food product. Craving a candy bar? Try eating a handful of nuts and a piece of fruit instead. Need a fast lunch? Try an avocado roll from the sushi cooler at the grocery store instead of a fast-food sandwich. The key is to choose a less processed food, not another heavily processed food product sporting a feel-good label.

MYTH #5: Modern medical treatments can fix your heart

> ➤ **The reality:** Unlike lifestyle medicine, which can heal your heart, modern medicine masks symptoms with dangerous drugs and invasive surgeries

Modern medicine is incredibly capable at reducing symptoms, but even the most advanced medications and procedures to relieve dangerously reduced heart function do not fix the problems with your heart.

Perhaps you're already taking prescription medication or have undergone invasive surgery after being diagnosed with heart disease. If so, you probably know the drill: First, doctors prescribe heart medicine that reduces cholesterol levels. That works for a few more heartbeats until the deposits build up even more, the drug having done nothing to solve the core problems that caused the dangerous buildup in the first place (problems we'll talk about in Part II). When the symptoms worsen, you undergo angioplasty, a procedure in which doctors push tubes, called catheters, through the system and pump them up to improve your blood flow. When the situation gets worse, they insert stents to hold the arteries open, and when it gets really bad, they build a new section of artery around the blockage (bypass surgery). These procedures do save people's lives and are done with incredible precision and admirable intentions—but they do nothing to solve the underlying problems.

One of the primary misconceptions about modern medical treatments for heart disease is that doctors can fix a damaged heart. On the contrary, research has proven that angioplasty, stenting, and bypass surgery, although they relieve symptoms, cannot repair the heart. This misconception has led many people to make poor lifestyle choices. Think of it this way: if you knew a mechanic couldn't fix your car and you couldn't ever buy a new one, wouldn't you take a little better care of it?

The reality is that a heart can only be fixed, and heart disease risk reduced, when internal inflammation is reduced and metabolic (energy conversion) balance restored, allowing the body's natural healing processes to do their thing. This can be done—I see my patients do it every day—and the Precision, Personalized Solution detailed in Part III will show you how.

Have you already been diagnosed with heart disease and advised to undergo a serious procedure? Or has your doctor suggested you start taking medications? Before you go to your next appointment, skip ahead to Chapter 9, where I walk you through specific questions to ask your doctor and when to ask them. If you do not have a heart disease diagnosis but are worried about your health and perhaps taking certain medications you'd like to leave behind, keep reading! You're holding in your hands a guide for truly repairing your heart. By the end of this book, your prognosis for heart health, as well as your quality of life, will be much brighter!

MYTH #6: Statin drugs are safe and will reduce heart attack risk for anyone who takes them

> ➤ **The reality:** Statin drugs cause serious issues for many people, many of which go unreported, and are largely ineffective in those who do not have heart disease

You already know from our comparison of Beth and Jenny and their cholesterol scores how statins can be ineffective at treating heart disease or preventing a heart attack. But perhaps even worse, statins are prescribed as if they are completely safe. They are not. Here's the real score on statins:

- Almost 9 percent of people on statin drugs—and as many as half of elderly women taking them—will become diabetic, and diabetes increases the risk of heart disease more in women than it does in men. One study examining hormone health in post-menopausal women evaluated the risks and benefits of statin drugs and found no benefit of stroke reduction and a 51 percent increased risk of diabetes.

- Because they deplete the antioxidant coenzyme Q^{10}, statins can cause mitochondrial poisoning, which reduces muscle function and leads as many as 18 percent of people on statin drugs to report muscle pain (and those are just the ones who feel the dysfunction and report it). Statins do reduce cholesterol levels, but reduced cholesterol levels are strongly linked to mood disorders, including depression. Recent research suggests that statins may induce depression, through the severe reduction of cholesterol levels, but contradictory evidence suggests that statin use is associated with a slight decrease in depression. (In my opinion, this slight decrease is probably due to the drug's anti-inflammatory qualities, not the reduced cholesterol; statins may help depression related to inflammation, but worsen depression related to reduced cholesterol.)

To understand just how few of the 25 million Americans on statin drugs really benefit from them, consider the drug's number needed to treat (NNT), a pharmacological tool to determine the effectiveness of a drug. The NNT is a calculation of how many people need to be treated with the drug for one person to have a certain benefit. The NNT score for drugs to prevent heart disease is usually the number of people who need to be treated in order to prevent one death. Plugging pharmaceutical cost per person into the equation allows this model to also be used to determine the cost of using the medicine to prevent a single death.

Another number that is critical to evaluating pharmaceuticals is the number needed to harm, or how many people must take the drug for one person to be harmed. Consideration of this number was a big part of my world when I was working on a master's degree in pharmacology.

For statin drugs, the NNT ranges vary depending on the particular drug, the patient's history of previous heart attacks or stroke, the dose, and patient age and gender. A study of women in the United Kingdom showed that for women younger than fifty, the NNT for statin drugs is 5,000. In other words, 5,000 forty-nine-year-old women would need to take statin drugs for the rest of their lives for just one of them to benefit! Other populations tell a different NNT story: 16 to 23 people who have already had heart attacks or strokes must take statins to prevent one death (in other words, the drug is far more beneficial for people who have already had a heart attack or stroke). For people of all ages and genders who have not had a heart incident, the NNT is between 250 and 500.

We must also take into account that 9 out of 100 people who take statins will become diabetic. Out of those 5,000 women under fifty who need to take statins to prevent one death, 450 will become diabetic. That's bad. The cost evaluation using the NNT is mind-blowing as well. For that same group of 5,000 women, the cost of the statin prescriptions to prevent one death would be $1.5 million per year.

One Australian study of 8,000 women between ages seventy-six and eighty-two found that the risk of new-onset diabetes ranged from 17 percent at the lowest statin dose to 51 percent at the highest. This means that for older people the number needed to harm is very low—at the high dose, more than half the people who take the drug will become diabetic. The number of people who suffer muscle damage from statin use is hard to quantify because much of it is never reported. Even if minor muscle damage is not noticed, however, it still reduces vitality.

One research paper explained the misunderstandings around statin drugs like this: "The benefits of these drugs are likely exaggerated, partly by an unconscious 'hope bias' on the part of readers and authors." If you're taking statins, you're undoubtedly hoping to be one of the people who benefit from them. However, if you're a forty-nine-year-old woman, does this hope of being the one in five thousand really make it worthwhile to take a drug that dramatically increases your chances of suffering muscle damage, diabetes, and maybe even depression? Especially when lifestyle medicine has proven to be so much more effective at preventing heart disease and improving quality of life than statins and can make life better for all five thousand women? Lifestyle medicine has proven to be equally effective at the one thing statins do best, reducing cholesterol, and so there is truly nothing statin drugs do better than lifestyle medicine.

Unfortunately, doctors are not trained to use this kind of NNT discussion to explain the efficacy of statin drugs to the public. Instead, they use data based on secondary trials, conducted with participants already diagnosed with coronary heart disease. The data gleaned from these trials make statins sound a lot more appealing, so doctors are trained to use this pitch instead: "Statins reduce participants' risk of death from heart attack by 30 percent." This number is wildly misleading because not only is it based on the people for whom statins are most beneficial, those who already have heart

NNT Chart

Drug	NNT Score	Context/Details
Antibiotic treatment for *H. pylori* bacteria to prevent recurrent stomach ulcer	2 (98 of 100 people treated benefit from the treatment)	No recurrence for a year (with additional medications used in the *H. pylori* cocktail)
Cholesterol-lowering statins for women younger than fifty with no history of heart disease	5,000 (5,000 women must take the drug to prevent one death)	• Nine in 100 people taking statins become diabetic • Forty to 50 percent increase for older women in the risk of developing diabetes from cholesterol medication • Women on statins have a higher risk of developing diabetes than men on statins • About one in ten people on statins suffer muscle damage In sum, treating 500 people with statins prevents one death and gives 50 to 250 of them diabetes, thus increasing their risk for a future heart attack
Cholesterol-lowering statins for women over fifty with no history of heart disease	500 (500 women must take the drug to prevent one death)	
Cholesterol-lowering statins for patients who have already been diagnosed with heart disease or had a heart attack	• 39 (39 must take the drug to prevent one nonfatal heart attack) • 83 (83 must take the drug to prevent one death from heart attack) • 125 (125 must take the drug to prevent one stroke)	
Cholesterol-lowering statins for women and men with risk factors such as diabetes or high blood pressure	250 (up to 250 must take the drug to prevent one heart attack or stroke)	
Cholesterol-lowering statins for women and men with no diagnosis of heart disease yet	500 (over 500 must take the drug to prevent one death from heart attack)	

disease, *but it is a 30 percent reduction in a percentage that was already very small.* For example, if three out of 100 people die *without* statins and two out of 100 people die *with* statins, this is a reduction of 33 percent. Nevertheless, 30 percent is the number doctors most often use to explain the benefit of statin drugs.

Besides presenting data in a way that makes statins look more effective than they really are, proponents of statins may also be giving them credit for a reduction in heart disease they had nothing to do with: for the general population, heart disease was most dramatically reduced during the time period before statins were invented. Although I do sometimes prescribe statins to my patients who are at extreme risk, I have come to a similar conclusion as the researchers who said, "We believe that lifestyle interventions such as the Mediterranean diet are substantially more powerful than statin medication in achieving cardiovascular benefits, and come without harms."

MYTH #7: Dieting is key to reversing heart disease

➤ **The reality:** Ping-pong dieting solely to lose weight can be even worse for heart health than excess pounds

Let's start with the whole notion of "diet"—a word I have banned from my clinic entirely (we use "personalized nutrition plan" instead)—and just look at the first three letters of the word: d-i-e!

Extremely low-fat and low-carbohydrate diets have both been known to cause problems with energy levels and mood and, true to the nature of anything extreme, are almost always bound to fail in the long run. This is why "diet"—defined as a short-term calorie restriction with the goal of losing weight—is indeed a four-letter word. In my clinic, I never prescribe a short-term diet, or any diet focused only on weight loss. For one, there is simply too much data supporting the dangers of dieting for weight loss. And second, if our goal is to balance the body's systems, then an extreme diet is counterproductive and probably increases inflammation and heart disease risk in the long run.

Today two distinctly different meanings of the word "diet" have emerged. One is the word's actual definition: what a person eats. The second is the one more often intended these days: eating less or differently in order to lose weight. Get this: by age five, the average girl's ideas about dieting are already formed based on her mother's dieting. Half of teenage girls have dieted in an attempt to change the shape of their bodies. And almost one-quarter of women with a normal body mass index (BMI)—weight-to-height ratio—still attempt to lose weight by dieting.

From paleo and Atkins to ketogenic and low-fat, dieting is a mess of overcomplicated fads and downright deception. There are a lot of forces at work persuading women to take dramatic steps to lose weight. After all, if you're overweight, losing weight is a good thing, right?

Obesity is so closely associated with heart disease that, for all practical purposes, it *is* heart disease. Obesity raises blood pressure, increases bad LDL cholesterol levels, and causes diabetes; conversely, a healthy body weight supports healthy blood pressure, balanced cholesterol levels, and healthy blood sugar control. Getting down to a healthy weight is certainly good for your heart—provided you can keep the weight off, preserve your energy levels and nutrition, and enjoy life in the process.

One of the worst things a woman can do, however, is yo-yo with her weight: Lose it, then put in back on. Lose it, then regain it. The data on this type of dieting are dismal. Ninety-five percent of women who lose 5 percent of their body weight regain it within nine years. But such body weight fluctuations are a proven risk factor for heart disease: some data have even shown that these fluctuations increase the risk of heart attack by 117 percent, and of stroke by 136 percent, compared to people with little body weight fluctuation. Radical body weight fluctuations may be even more damaging to the heart than staying obese! By contrast, when my patients lose weight as a side effect of heart-healing lifestyle medicine, the weight tends to stay off, and they may even continue to optimize their weight many years after initiating the program.

My patient Meredith is one of the best examples of how dieting, in its modern sense, can cause problems. Meredith came to see me in 2010 for a smorgasbord of issues, including heart problems, but also irritable bowel syndrome (IBS), dry skin and brittle hair, poor sleep, anxiety, and fatigue. She was also suffering from excess weight and type 2 diabetes and had experimented with strict, food-specific "diets."

One of the first things I did was give Meredith a blood test for food sensitivity. "When I saw the results," she recalls, "I hyperventilated." Meredith's system was sensitive to a number of foods that she was eating nearly every day, so she was bombarding her system with an inflammatory immune response at every meal, despite being on a "healthy diet." She replaced those foods with others that provided the same nutrition and also began taking a few high-quality targeted supplements. Within six months, Meredith's top five complaints were 90 percent resolved, her blood pressure was down, and her hormone balance and thyroid levels were improved.

In a follow-up interview seven years later, Meredith said happily, "They're all fixed; my whole body is better!" In another of those double-edged swords of health, dieting was partly responsible for her problems, but building an every-day-for-a-lifetime personalized nutrition plan based on her unique food sensitivities, nutrient deficiencies, hormone imbalances, inflammation and toxicity levels, and nutritional needs formed the solution to her problems. (In Part II, we'll do a deep dive into inflammation, hormones, toxicity, and more, and in Chapter 6, you'll learn all about pairing your unique food sensitivities with proper food.)

As Meredith demonstrated so wonderfully, the only way around this minefield is for women who care about their heart health to be their own greatest advocates. And one of the most important things a woman can do to become her own advocate is to not fall into the trap of dieting for weight loss alone. Make weight loss a side effect of a nutrition plan and a lifestyle designed to heal, however, and you're on your way to optimal health. When weight loss accompanies healing, a third—and perhaps the best—definition of the word "diet" emerges: *making food choices that benefit health.*

Even though I may not like the word and usually avoid recommending any packaged diet, I understand that you may feel that a structured "diet" suits your decision-making methods best. In that case, it's probably best to choose a personalized nutrition plan that borrows the key elements of the Mediterranean diet: whole-grain carbohydrates, healthy oils, small servings of high-quality protein such as fish and grass-fed meat, fruits and vegetables, all consumed in the company of people you love. Besides data that suggests the Mediterranean diet may dramatically reduce death from all causes, the food choices are also appetizing enough to be sustained over a lifetime, a benefit that probably has contributed to its rise to the top of diet fads. But it's still a diet, and the studies that showed this highly publicized diet to be so beneficial are now under fire for unscrupulous scientific process. This doesn't mean the diet isn't beneficial, but just how beneficial is in question—it might even be more beneficial than the numbers suggest . . .

Better than any diet, a personalized nutrition plan is a framework for making decisions based on your individual health baseline and an understanding of how your particular body reacts to the inflammatory potential of your food. One of the greatest benefits of this approach is that it allows you to be flexible with the different cuisines you encounter while you're traveling, enjoying the holidays, or eating dinner with friends—in other words, to enjoy life while also bolstering your vascular health and preventing heart disease. And I'll help you design this personalized nutrition plan in Part III.

Find Your Icaria

As Meredith discovered, for anyone who does their homework to determine what their unique body needs, there is no one-stop shop that once found will eliminate the need for daily decision-making and ongoing, conscious management of health. The solution becomes an ever-changing part of who you are, not an end point that you arrive at where you never have to think about health again. I always say that I'm a doctor in moderation—meaning, if you slip every once in a while, I think that's okay. It's better to embrace being imperfect and continue doing the best you can than to give up on optimal heart health and vitality because you find it impossible to be perfect. The solution is found in striving for improved health every day, because the alternative—continuing blindly toward disease and lower vitality—has perhaps the worst consequence of all: a less enjoyable life.

Think of it this way: even those people living in regions with the healthiest lifestyles on the planet succumb to modern ailments when they leave their homeland. For example, the Icarians, who live on the Greek island of Icaria off the coast of Turkey, became famous after the National Geographic "Blue Zone" project, which set out to discover the world's longest-lived populations. Icarians have half the US rate of cardiovascular disease, 20 percent less cancer, almost no dementia or Alzheimer's, and they are three times more likely than Americans to live to see ninety. On their island, Icarians take a daily nap, frequently connect with friends, and eat a plant-based diet supplemented with plenty of olive oil, whole grains, and fish. But when Icarians leave Icaria, their risk of cardiovascular disease, cancer, and dementia rises to the same level as that found in the country they emigrate to!

Nobody has done this study yet, but it would be telling to transplant 100 Americans at high risk for heart disease to Icaria and see how they do for the next few decades. My money would be on those people doing much better than people with similar risk factors back in America.

The solution to heart disease prevention—and many other diseases for that matter—is found in creating your own personal Icaria. When you create your own island of health and longevity in a sea of inflammation and disease potential, you can take it with you wherever you go, just as Meredith did. Creating this island is economical and achievable, and you're almost ready to start doing it. There is just one more piece of the puzzle to consider before crafting your Precision, Personalized Solution: the powerful synergy between the heart, brain, gut, and genes. Now, in Part II, you'll learn about how the body uses information in the form of hormones to create a symphony of messaging that is either out of tune and slipping toward conditions where disease can take hold, or in tune and functioning smoothly to prevent, resist, and even reverse disease.

Part II

Your Body and Disease

Chapter 3

Inflammation

The Root Cause of Disease

My extensive work with patients suffering from declining vascular function corroborates what the vast research on it has finally revealed is the root cause of heart disease. It's not the buildup of cholesterol. It's not animal fats clogging our arteries. It's not the result of choosing Wendy's over Subway or Coke Classic over Diet Coke. Rather, the root cause of heart disease is inflammation, in the form of hormonal and genetic messaging that increases the inflammatory molecules circulating in the bloodstream and passing through the heart along with the 100 gallons of blood it pumps each day. These inflammatory molecules include the insulin and other amino acids and proteins from our metabolic processes as well as defensive antigens from our immune response. Insulin is essential for converting blood sugar into energy, but it is also the most inflammatory molecule your body makes. This is why sugars, sodas, and even bread and bagels cause blood sugar spikes that light the fire of inflammation then pour the metaphorical gas of insulin all over it.

The activity of these inflammatory molecules wears down your heart prematurely. By causing the intestinal barriers to become more permeable (which you'll learn more about in Chapter 5), inflammation allows the passage of more unwanted particles into the bloodstream. This incites additional inflammation and immune response. Over time, this inflammatory reaction wears down the inner lining of the arteries, and the result is atherosclerosis (hardening of the arteries), which ages your heart prematurely.

Inflammation's destructive activity doesn't stop there. Emerging evidence suggests that inflammation is a primary driver in the development of not only heart disease but also dementia, cancer, depression, chronic fatigue, fibromyalgia, irritable bowel disease, and more. Inflammation also reduces the body's ability to process the chemicals and toxins we are exposed to daily and sabotages our hormones, making us feel sick and tired.

Inflammation is the primary driver of disease in general, and heart disease specifically. If you have a heart disease diagnosis, you are suffering from chronic inflammation. If you have diabetes or obesity and feel you are at high risk for developing heart disease, you are also suffering from inflammation. If you have asthma, eczema, arthritis, acne, regular bloating or discomfort, stubborn weight, even afternoon energy slumps and insatiable cravings—you are likely suffering from unnecessarily high or unregulated amounts of inflammation in your body. When it becomes chronic, inflammation causes disease.

Inflammation has been in the news a lot lately, so much so that, if you're interested enough in your own vitality and health to be reading this book, you've probably already heard about it. You may know by now that increasing inflammation in your body's system decreases your health and moves your body closer to disease and, conversely, that reducing inflammation in your body's systems makes you healthier overall and encourages your body's incredible natural healing ability to resist and even reverse chronic disease.

The tricky part isn't understanding that inflammation can contribute to disease and that reducing inflammation makes you healthier.

This makes perfect sense. The tricky part is figuring out what part of *your* life causes inflammation in *your* body.

It's an intimidating (and intriguing) challenge, but you are the most qualified person in the world to take it on, and this book will help you do that. After helping thousands of women find the inflammatory causes in their own lives—and learning that women are very, very good at knowing what's bothering them—I am pretty certain that if you list the things in your normal day that might cause inflammation (particularly after reading this chapter), you'll come up with a much more accurate list of your inflammation sources than any doctor, no matter how many letters they have behind their name.

To get a picture of how inflammation invades and throws off the balance of the body, let's follow a fictional day in the life of a woman named Claire, who cares deeply about her life, her health, and her loved ones. Claire has a demanding career, is raising an active family, enjoys a couple of hobbies, and, although not perfectly content with some aspects of her life, figures she has it pretty darn good in the grand scheme of things. Maybe Claire is nothing like you, but for this one chapter, put yourself in her shoes, her mind-set, and her place in life. In subsequent chapters, I'll help you look more closely at the inflammatory triggers in the *real* you.

Morning

The inflammatory day starts early and ends late, and it usually has something to do with a baby. Your "baby" may not be your actual offspring. For some of us, the baby is a career. For others, the baby is a hobby. Or a pet. Maybe a partner. Of course, for many of us the baby is an actual child.

Our babies give us something to live for—they motivate us and inspire us to make good decisions. The problem is, when you have a baby, it is all too easy to let old number one—you—take second place. Or third. Or fourth.

Claire's babies are her family and her work. She has a son and a daughter, both in elementary school. Her work is sort of a necessary evil—not exactly inspiring, but it pays the bills. Both her work and her family bump Claire far down on the priority list. For the sake of our goal here to reverse and resist heart disease while improving overall vitality and quality of life, let's focus on the little things—the many decisions Claire makes every day that seem small and insignificant in the moment but that have very real consequences for her internal balance and the health of her heart.

When Claire wakes up in the morning, the first thing she thinks about is everything she has to do to take care of her babies. The kids need breakfast made and lunches packed. She needs to make sure they brush their teeth and pack their homework. If her daughter is having a bad hair day, complete with tears and tantrums, Claire has to spend time helping her daughter wrestle the tangles from her hair instead of making herself a real breakfast. Once the kids are out the door, Claire's attention shifts quickly and purposefully to taking care of her work baby. She tosses her children's dishes in the dishwasher on her way out the door, grabs the half-a-bagel-and-cream-cheese her son left sitting on his plate, and downs the rest of his orange juice. She wraps the bagel in a napkin to eat on the commute and, knowing that a bagel isn't the most nutritious food, grabs a granola bar for an easy and "healthy" breakfast complement.

Claire munches the granola bar and sips a coffee out of a to-go mug in the madhouse morning traffic while listening to the day's news and her favorite podcast. The news is the usual combination of dysfunctional politics, stomach-churning disasters halfway around the world, and traffic updates that, even in the absence of delays on her own route, put her on edge, making her anxious to get to the office, get out of the car, check her email, and settle into her day.

The Stress Response

Let's stop here and unpack what just happened. The events of Claire's day have already put her system into stress mode by early morning. Between the frenzy of getting the family out the door, traffic, and the downright awful daily news that is somehow both nauseating and irresistible, Claire is already experiencing inflammatory biochemical processes burning inside her in the form of her stress response. Her body's most vocal messengers—her hormones—are responding to the events of the day so far with the ancient fury of an animal in danger. In other words, her endocrine system is flooding her body with stress hormones, including dopamine, epinephrine (better known as adrenaline), prolactin, and cortisol.

This cocktail of hormones works with the nervous system to activate your ancestral fight-or-flight response—which is good for saving a child from a burning car or escaping from a flooding river, but terribly detrimental as part of your daily routine. To help you clamber out of the raging torrent, dopamine increases your blood pressure, which gives your muscles a boost of oxygen. Epinephrine triggers your blood to release adenosine triphosphate (ATP), the currency of the body's energy system. This chemical form of energy is exchanged rapidly between cells. The epinephrine-induced ATP release is like the president declaring a national disaster in order to access emergency funding—an ATP release engages the full might of the body's energy potential. At the same time, cortisol, sometimes called the stress hormone, gives you an additional burst of energy, increased immunity, a reduced sensitivity to pain, and heightened mental awareness.

When your fight-or-flight response is activated by a traumatic event that requires your body's ultimate capabilities, you want every boost your system can muster. You want the blast of oxygen, the emergency energy funding, the natural pain killer, and the mental edge. But this superhero state is *expensive*. Afterwards, you want this entire physiological superhero state to end so you can go back to being your normal

The Endocrine System

Think of the endocrine system as the body's version of the internet, a cellular phone, the spoken word, smoke signals, and sign language, all making up the internal communication system that functions separately from the nervous system. The endocrine system allows the glands to talk to each other using a system so complex that even the most advanced science is far from revealing precisely how it all works. The method of communication used by the endocrine system has been referred to in physiology textbooks as "wireless," meaning that its components (glands and organs) are not directly connected to each other structurally with tissues or nerves. The nervous system differs from the endocrine system in that the messages of the nervous system travel along the "wiring" of neural connections.

The endocrine system uses hormones released into the blood to send messages across the body and between cells. In comparison to the nervous system, which functions at lightning speed with response time measured in milliseconds, the endocrine system generally operates much more slowly, requiring seconds, minutes, and sometimes days or even longer to transmit messages. This is why problems originating in the endocrine system can be so difficult to pinpoint: by the time we suffer the consequences of the dysfunction caused by hormonal messaging, the influence that caused the damaging messages to be sent often is long gone. The slower time frame of hormonal messaging also allows one message to build on top of another, creating a super-size and extremely complex wave of influence that can have far-reaching, significant, and seemingly disconnected consequences.

self and allow your system to recover. Unfortunately for Claire, since her life has been stressful for some time, her body is in a constant state of Wonder Woman—or tries to be.

The problem is that her body, like yours and mine, is simply not designed to sustain the superhero response over time, so the physical response to stress changes dramatically as the source of the stress goes from a short-term emergency to the everyday norm. After her prolonged stress response, Claire's body can no longer convert fats and sugars into ATP molecules to burn as energy, so it does the next best thing: it converts the sugar to fat and stores it. *This is why chronic stress causes weight gain.* On top of weight gain, a reduced ATP response has been associated with fatigue, depression, reduced immunity, insomnia, and other serious health issues.

Then there's the cortisol. Prolonged high levels of this stress hormone have been associated with decreases in immunity, bone density, and muscle tissue, as well as reduced thyroid and mental function. Cortisol also increases blood pressure and over time contributes to blood sugar imbalance and the storage of visceral fat surrounding the organs—the most damaging fat in your body.

Perhaps worst of all, the prolonged stress response has been associated with reducing the body's ability to manage the inflammatory response. Research shows clearly that people with chronic stress have elevated levels of inflammation and an increase in rates of heart disease, depression, autoimmune disease, respiratory infections, and even poor wound healing.

Sugar with Your Sugar

I'm sure you can see where this is going for Claire. Not only has her stress response been activated by morning traffic and the hassle of getting the kids out the door, but she has created a double attack on her internal balance with her hasty carbohydrate- and sugar-fueled breakfast. When we think about stress, we usually picture it as arising from circumstances beyond our control—Claire's daughter's tangled hair and inevitable tears, for example. That kind of stressful moment may trigger an inflammatory stress response in Claire, but that inflammation is normal and our bodies are built to endure and recover quickly from such moments. All too often in our chaotic modern world, however, it's not the singular and passing stresses that make inflammation "systemic" or "chronic," but rather the choices we make. For Claire it's the bagel, orange juice, and granola bar fueling the fire and preventing her hormonal messaging from dousing the flames of her stress response.

Let's start with the granola bar, one of thousands of products sold as "health food" that are hardly better than junk food and in fact even poison to some people. For Claire, the granola bar contains several troublemakers.

Here's the ingredient list from a popular granola bar:

GRANOLA (WHOLE GRAIN ROLLED OATS, BROWN SUGAR, CRISP RICE [RICE FLOUR, SUGAR, SALT, MALTED BARLEY EXTRACT], WHOLE GRAIN ROLLED WHEAT, SOYBEAN OIL, WHOLE WHEAT FLOUR, SODIUM BICARBONATE, SOY LECITHIN, CARAMEL COLOR, NONFAT DRY MILK), CORN SYRUP, BROWN RICE CRISP (WHOLE GRAIN BROWN RICE, SUGAR, MALTED BARLEY FLOUR, SALT), PEANUT BUTTER SPREAD (PEANUTS, SUGAR, PALM OIL, SALT), SEMISWEET CHOCOLATE CHIPS (SUGAR, CHOCOLATE LIQUOR, COCOA BUTTER, SOY LECITHIN, VANILLA EXTRACT), INVERT SUGAR, PEANUT FLAVORED CHIPS (SUGAR, PALM KERNEL AND PALM OIL, PARTIALLY DEFATTED PEANUT FLOUR, LACTOSE, DRY WHEY, DEXTROSE, CORN SYRUP SOLIDS, SOY LECITHIN, SALT, VANILLIN [ARTIFICIAL FLAVOR]), CORN SYRUP SOLIDS, GLYCERIN. CONTAINS 2% OR LESS OF CALCIUM CARBONATE, SORBITOL, SALT, WATER, NATURAL AND ARTIFICIAL FLAVOR, BHT (PRESERVATIVE), CITRIC ACID.

This ingredient list mentions sugar no less than ten times. You already know from Chapter 2 about the connection between sugar intake and heart disease. The first ingredient is granola, but sugar is the second ingredient in the granola. Corn syrup (more sugar) is the fourth ingredient. Brown rice crisp has sugar as a second ingredient. Then come the semisweet chocolate chips and peanut-flavored chips (both with sugar as their first ingredient). After that, there's corn syrup solids (different from corn syrup, but still sugar as far as your heart health is concerned).

Making matters worse, to Claire's metabolism (how she uses energy), the simple carbohydrates in the bagel and the rice in the granola bar are also sugar. The way the human body processes simple carbohydrates may seem to defy common sense, but in fact there's a significant difference between complex and simple carbohydrates. Whole-wheat flour and brown rice are slow-to-digest complex carbohydrates, but fiber, a critical element of the grain—and an element that our bodies evolved to use in digestion—is removed when they're processed into white flour and white rice. Removing the fiber makes white flour and white rice light and fluffy, but it also makes the resulting simple carbohydrate incredibly quick to digest. The blood sugar difference between simple and complex carbohydrates is a little like the difference between drinking a glass of wine on an empty stomach versus a glass with a hearty dinner. On the empty stomach, the alcohol goes straight to your head and leaves you spinning, while drinking the same glass with dinner slows your body's alcohol absorption because it's busy processing food along with it and the narcotic effect is much reduced. This is why fiber is so beneficial: it slows the process of digestion.

The slow digestion of complex carbohydrates allows your body to convert food into energy at a pace that doesn't overload your bloodstream with sugar. This slow-burn carbohydrate is the kind of carbohydrate the human body digested for thousands of years until the modern industrial food machine was built and flooded our world with simple carbohydrates. (In Chapter 6, page 206, I list some of my favorite complex carbohydrates that can be enjoyed throughout the day.) The human body is simply not optimized to consume large quantities of simple carbohydrates. From the body's point of view, there is little difference between eating sugar and eating white flour.

In fact, white flour bombards the bloodstream with sugar even faster than table sugar. Here's how:

When Claire bites into that bagel, the food triggers her brain to release saliva from three pairs of large salivary glands and hundreds of smaller glands located around the lining of the mouth. Before she even swallows, enzymes in her saliva have already begun to digest the carbohydrates in the bagel—the first step in converting the carbohydrates into glucose (ready-to-be-burned sugar) for her body to use for energy.

After she swallows, her stomach walls churn the chewed food into a pulp called chyme. Digestive juices further break down the chyme and prepare it for the nutritional shopping center of the small intestine. Within fifteen minutes of taking those first bites—about the time it takes her to eat the bagel and the granola bar—her digestive juices have already converted the simple carbohydrates of the bagel into glucose. This means that, by the time the bagel reaches her small intestine, it's essentially sugar. It also means that the granola bar, which already contained ten sugars, is now accompanied by a whole lot more sugar.

The Glycemic Index

The glycemic index (GI) is a scale from 1 to 100 that gives a relative value for how much a particular food will affect your blood sugar levels. A plain, white bagel is a 95 on the GI, while a Coca-Cola is a 63—in other words, eating that plain white bagel spikes your blood sugar levels faster than drinking a Coke!

Perhaps even more shocking, the glycemic index reveals that a glass of fruit juice, like the orange juice Claire quickly drank before heading out the door, produces a spike in blood sugar similar to a Coke (OJ ranges between 50 and 76 on the GI scale). Sure, the juice may have additional vitamins and minerals in it (if it's high-quality, fresh juice), and it's devoid of Coke's myriad artificial ingredients and caffeine, but the impact of juice and Coke on your metabolism and sugar load—and thus your heart health—is essentially the same. This is an earth-shaking realization. Chugging that glass of orange juice may

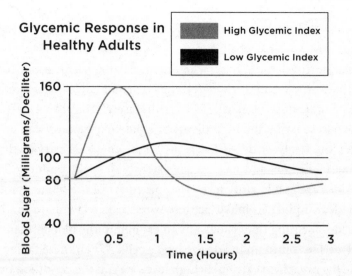

Glycemic Response in Healthy Adults

High Glycemic Index

Low Glycemic Index

have felt to Claire like a healthy thing to do; a health-conscious person like her never would have pounded a Coke in the same scenario. As it turns out, neither is good for her—or for you.

When you consume simple carbohydrates (say, a glass of fruit juice or a cinnamon roll), your blood sugar spikes up and then drops, leaving you in a low blood sugar state that we call the "sugar blues" starting about ninety minutes after you finish that roll. But when you add protein, you blunt that trajectory: your blood sugar doesn't spike quite as high, or drop quite as low.

So if orange juice is bad for us, why are orange slices still considered healthy? When we eat the whole fruit, the fiber in the fruit dramatically slows the flow of sugar into the bloodstream, just as the fiber in complex carbohydrates like whole grains slow the transformation of carbohydrates into blood sugar. When we drink the juice alone, the sugar gets the fast track to the bloodstream. It takes about eight oranges to make a 16-ounce glass of orange juice. When was the last time you tried to eat eight oranges with breakfast? The fiber of the orange not only fills you up but also slows both your consumption and digestion of the sugar, allowing your liver to process the sugar at a pace it can handle. Once your blood sugar levels exceed a certain amount, your liver treats the sugar as a toxin (rightfully so!) and packages it up in the form of angry, inflammatory, hard-to-burn visceral fat. This fat is then stored around your organs and midsection—arguably the worst fat in the universe when it comes to heart health.

Besides storing fat, the liver, when metabolizing sugar, produces triglycerides—three bad, sticky fatty acids that, at high levels, are one of the key indicators of elevated heart disease risk. When I use a centrifuge to separate the ingredients of a patient's blood, I can actually see the triglycerides if levels are high. They're a part of the blood that looks like, and has the consistency of, sticky pudding. If triglycerides are at a healthy level, the same part of the blood spins out as a clear liquid. To make matters worse, when there are more triglycerides forming than the liver can expel into the bloodstream, the triglycerides build up inside the liver's cells. When these fat levels in the liver reach an extremely high level, we call the condition by the not-so-appetizing term "fatty liver." The vascular damage caused by excessive sugar and simple carbohydrate consumption is, in my opinion, a key player in our current epidemics of obesity, diabetes, and poor heart health.

I know it's a bit depressing. The last few pages, and much of today's health news, probably make you feel like no matter what you eat or do, you're not doing the right thing. That only adds to the stress. Just writing about the effects of sugar and simple carbs makes me want to eat a cookie and give up on vitality and health. But before you throw in the towel, let me share a bit of good news that will give you just an inkling of the food and lifestyle medicine yet to come in *Heart Solution for Women*: when mice are fed enough sugar to cause fatty liver disease, the condition can be reversed by giving the mice derivatives of kefir, the fermented yogurt drink found in many grocery stores. The amino acids and microbes in kefir (and other fermented foods) are powerful medicine. When these same mice are given supplements of amino acids derived from kefir, their fatty liver symptoms decline, their inflammation indicator markers go down, the indicators associated with diabetes, including insulin resistance and glucose tolerance, improve, and they show decreased weight gain even as overall calorie consumption remains the same. If one simple change can provide this much benefit, imagine what a multifaceted

The Role of Insulin

Insulin is a delivery hormone that attaches itself to blood sugar and opens the door to a cell so that the cell can use the glucose as energy. As blood sugar levels increase, the body produces more insulin in an attempt to use the sugar. When the cells have used all the glucose they need but continue to be bombarded by glucose-carrying insulin, over time the cells become insulin-resistant: they stop opening the door when insulin knocks, even when they need the energy. Insulin resistance increases blood sugar levels, decreases energy levels, and increases sugar conversion to fat, a trilogy of dysfunction you (and your heart) definitely don't want.

A glucose tolerance test is a measure of insulin function used to determine how well the body is utilizing insulin. In this test, a sugary drink is consumed and then measures are taken of how quickly the sugar dissipates (is absorbed by the cells). In a body with insulin resistance, the cells do not absorb the sugar and the sugar levels remain elevated. In a body with healthy insulin and blood sugar control, the sugar levels will decline quickly as the cells open their doors and absorb the sugar.

solution designed for you, with your specific needs in mind, will do to reduce your heart disease risk and increase your quality of life!

Now you know more about nutrition than I did upon graduating from medical school, and we haven't even gotten to Claire's lunch yet.

Midday

By the time lunch break rolls around, Claire has endured a Mount Everest–high blood sugar spike and a Death Valley–low crash. Munching a dark chocolate bar she had stashed in her desk for the midmorning slump kept her going; besides, she's heard that dark chocolate is good for women. Unfortunately, because of all the sugar added to dark chocolate to make it sweet and the extensive processing that destroys most of the delicate flavonoids—the plant nutrient found in cocoa that is responsible for the supposed health benefits of chocolate—most dark chocolate, unless it's more than about 75 percent cocoa, is no better for blood sugar balance than any other candy with similar sugar content. Claire's chocolate bar of choice, even though it says "dark chocolate" on the package, contains only 45 percent cocoa.

It's been a great quarter in Claire's company, so her boss invites the team to a steakhouse for lunch. After her meager breakfast and busy morning, she orders an eight-ounce sirloin for herself.

The Meat Dilemma

Meat can be part of a healthy diet, but unless it's the right kind of meat at the right quantity, it comes at a price to heart health. That price is especially high when the meat is the kind of factory-raised, corn-fed, hormone-antibiotic-steroid-injected beef Claire just ordered.

For the moment, let's forget about the quality of the beef and consider what your body does with protein. Unlike carbohydrates, proteins don't begin to break down in the mouth. It takes the powerful hydrochloric acid in the stomach, the action of the small intestine, and finally the nutrient-production workhorse in the liver to break down protein into the amino acids that your body can use to build and rebuild every structure in the body, from muscles to skin to the cells of our organs.

While waiting for the meal, Claire's boss, who ordered elk medallions, goes on a rant about how vegetarians are missing critical nutrition because of the lack of meat in their diet. The conversation reminds Claire of a conversation she had over the holidays with her sister, a vegetarian, who said that meat is bad because of the cholesterol and fat. As it turns out, neither Claire's boss nor her sister has it quite right.

Vegetarians can get all their needed nutrients from a meat-free diet if they make sure to eat enough of the right kinds of protein and fats. And meat does indeed contain elements that, particularly when consumed in large quantities, damage the vascular system. When an amino acid called methionine is metabolized, the chemical homocysteine is produced. I tell my patients that homocysteine is like a toxic protein that goes around chewing on your intima, the inner layer of your arteries, damaging this layer, and causing your body to send cholesterol to repair the damage. Precisely how homocysteine damages the intima, and whether it is a direct cause or a by-product of arterial damage is not entirely understood, but elevated homocysteine levels in the blood are very clearly associated with heart damage.

Methionine is considered an essential amino acid in the growth of blood vessels, but it's not only found in meat—it is also found in seaweed and sesame seeds. Methionine supplements are actually helpful against certain chronic diseases. In other words, methionine is not something that should or can be avoided, but rather an example of the importance of moderation in consumption of meat (as in so many other things). The homocysteine story also gives us another glimpse into the power of supplements: homocysteine levels can be reduced by taking vitamin B12 and folate supplements, which you'll learn more about in Chapter 8.

But what about that cholesterol in meat? This brings us once again to one of the most common misunderstandings in the world of food and health. As we touched on in the previous chapter, homocysteine and a gang of other prime suspects have been letting cholesterol take the rap for heart disease for the last forty years, but a new understanding of cardiovascular processes has lifted the curtain on the inflammatory effects of high levels of blood sugar and the arterial trauma of inflammation. Cholesterol isn't completely innocent, but it probably deserved only a few community service hours rather than forty years of hard time.

I always tell my patients that it's not the meat that causes the problems, but what's *in* the meat. And again, the steakhouse sirloin is not the only culprit. Most likely, any factory-farmed beef you buy from your neighborhood grocery store or order in a restaurant is a dye-coated, xenoestrogen-filled, highly inflammatory, omega-6 piece of meat.

Say what, you ask? Well, let me explain. Most supermarket meat is dyed with carbon monoxide to make it look bright red, even after it begins to age. If you've ever seen an animal butchered or been to a meat market outside of the United States, you know that meat isn't the color of a Christmas tree ornament—and it certainly doesn't stay that way after a couple of days. But the artificial coloring is one of the more benign aspects of factory-raised meat.

Xenoestrogens are the synthetic growth hormones fed to or injected into animals to increase meat, egg, and dairy production. They are the reason why the supermarket's industrially produced chicken breasts are the size of your foot while the organic chicken breasts are the size of your palm. These chemicals, which mimic human hormones, are passed to humans when we consume meat and act as what's called an endocrine disruptor—or a monkey wrench in your own hormones. When Claire digs into that industrially raised steak, she's giving herself a dose of synthetic female hormones that have been proven to increase the risk of cancer and other health problems. In young girls, xenoestrogens are associated with earlier puberty. Unfortunately, these chemicals have become so common that it's now nearly impossible for researchers to find control subjects who do not have them present in their bodily fluids. Xenoestrogens are yet another reason to optimize your internal balance every chance you get—the world bombards you with insults you can't control, so you might as well eliminate those you can control and bolster your natural healing ability to handle the inevitable damage that is part and parcel of modern life on earth.

Then there are the antibiotics given to livestock to manage illness in the horrid living conditions of factory farms. Seventy percent of all antibiotics produced in the world are given to livestock. The use of hormones and antibiotics in livestock is the reason why America, land of some of the most beautiful open spaces and forage-rich ranches on the planet, produces some of the world's worst meat. Much of the livestock raised on these gorgeous ranches will produce meat that is healthy to eat until it is taken to the feedlot and injected with hormones and antibiotics and fattened up with corn. (Consider this: the European Union will import only American beef that is certified to have no added hormones.)

The fatty acid omega-6 is another troublesome element in Claire's sirloin. You've probably heard of omega-3 fatty acids. Before I tell you more, it's useful to know that grass-fed beef has two to five times more omega-3 than grain-fed beef, and both types of beef contain omega-6.

Both omega-3 and omega-6 are essential fatty acids that we must get from our environment; they are not manufactured in our bodies like many other essential compounds, such as cholesterol. In the ideal body, omega-3 and omega-6 are found in relatively equal amounts. There's an easy way to understand how the balance of these two fatty acids is maintained: omega-6 stimulates inflammation for immune response, and omega-3 curbs the inflammatory immune response. Think of these fatty acids as your body's commanding generals. Your omega-6 sends out the troops and your omega-3 brings them home. Both are equally important for defense, but the problem is that the average Western diet is extremely heavy in omega-6 and dismally low in omega-3. Our omega-6 consumption is typically ten times higher than our omega-3 consumption. Ideally, we'd have an omega-6 to omega-3 ratio closer to two-to-one, or even one-to-one, but certainly not ten-to-one. With a ten-to-one ratio, we're really good at deploying the troops and firing up the inflammation but have a really hard time ending the conflict and bringing them home.

Claire's body has plenty of reasons to activate its defenses and send out the troops, but her body's ability to call off the attack is compromised by a poor omega-6 to omega-3 balance. Besides regulating inflammation, omega-3s are also essential for selective blood clotting and building cellular membranes in the brain. Studies have shown that people who eat fish weekly or who have higher levels of a particular type of omega-3 have a lower risk of developing dementia. For heart disease, omega-3 verges on the miraculous: omega-3 might even beat cholesterol-lowering drugs at their own game, is far more cost-effective, and carries no potential for muscle damage and other dangers. I'll share my recommendations for how to get these incredible omega-3s into your body in Chapter 6.

There's something else people don't think about when they consume large amounts of meat: eating meat puts a very real and immediate stress on the heart. If you're healthy, your body can handle that stress in small amounts, but if you were to take a brachial artery tourniquet test to measure your vasospasms (a sudden narrowing of the arteries) after eating a steak, it would show that you're still experiencing vasospasms for up to six hours. I've had patients with heart issues call me after leaving the steakhouse to complain of chest pains. They have to take a nitroglycerine tablet to reduce the vasospasms and make the pain go away. Why are they in pain? Because when their arteries are already irritable from chronic inflammation, vasospasms hurt.

If you're going to eat steak, spend the extra money to buy wild game or grass-fed meat that wasn't corn-finished in the feedlot, spiked with hormones, and loaded with antibiotics. You'll save the money later in medical bills.

Claire's vascular system is young enough, and strong enough, that she doesn't feel the vasospasms, but she returns to the office with even more inflammation in her body. If she had opted for a salmon salad, or the elk medallions her boss chose, she would have helped her body recover from a morning of inflammation with a nutritious anti-inflammatory gift. Instead, the sirloin steak created a new problem for her body to deal with. One of the incredible things you'll learn more about in Part III is how small changes can soothe inflammation and move you further away from the specter of disease.

The inflammation of the first half of Claire's day would have been significantly reduced if she had breakfasted on oatmeal with berries for sweetness instead of a granola bar, an orange instead of orange juice, and a whole-wheat bagel (or better yet, as I'll explain shortly, a gluten-free bagel) instead of a white flour bagel, followed by a pasture-raised steak instead of a factory-raised steak at lunch. And none of these food choices would have compromised flavor, food preference, or social engagement.

The Weekend Exerciser

After work, Claire drives home feeling guilty for skipping a gym session, breaking a New Year's resolution she made just six weeks earlier. But how could she have a good gym session, she rationalizes, when she's still sore from yesterday's bike ride? Since Claire had been slacking on exercise, she wanted to make up for it with a really long ride. The weather was beautiful, she had a tail wind on the way out, and she was feeling great. But when she turned around, the wind was in her face, her energy crashed, and she struggled to get back home. By the time she finally got off her bike, she could barely walk. But exercise is healthy, right?

As it turns out, exercise causes inflammation too. Like so many things in the ongoing battle to reduce inflammation, the difference between exercise that increases inflammation overall and exercise that decreases inflammation overall is difficult to measure. And more importantly, it's personal.

If each week Claire had been going to the gym a couple of days and riding her bike or going for a brisk walk several other days, as she resolved to do on January 1, that hard bike ride would indeed have reduced inflammation throughout her body, reduced her oxidative stress (caused by the burning of energy, oxidative stress is a primary driver of age-related decay), and made her heart and vascular system healthier. But because she hadn't been getting her heart rate up through regular exercise, only doing the occasional hard workout, the exertion caused her arteries to become inflamed. It also stressed her mitochondria—the energy factories of the muscles—to exert more than they were accustomed to, increasing the oxidative stress of energy conversion. The worst consequence of all, however, was that overdoing exercise over the weekend made physical exertion so unappealing that she made excuses to avoid additional exercise all week. By the next weekend, she will feel guilty enough that she'll go out and overdo it once more.

Where the difference lies between an inflammatory factor that contributes to disease and an anti-inflammatory healing factor that helps your body resist disease is unique to your particular body. One study demonstrated that a strenuous thirty-minute exercise session reduces oxidative stress and enhances arterial elasticity (both key components of a healthy heart), while a strenuous sixty-minute exercise session worsens oxidative stress and increases arterial stiffness. Not what you want. But after twenty years of working with athletes, I'm pretty sure that the people who exercised for sixty minutes in this study were not accustomed to exercise, because in fact frequent exercise increases cellular antioxidant ability. If the study participants exercised frequently before the study, sixty minutes of strenuous exercise would almost certainly have been at least as beneficial to them as the thirty-minute exercise. For Claire, the same bike ride that caused excessive inflammation would have been therapeutic if she had worked up to that level with bike rides or moderate exertion almost every day.

In Part III, you'll learn more about what types of exercise you need and what types to avoid or to skip. You'll learn what happens inside your vascular system when you exercise, why it is single-handedly the best tool you have for healing your heart, and how to exercise so that it is a refreshing and anti-inflammatory part of your day rather than a difficult, inflammatory, and even demoralizing ordeal. What's most exciting is that exercise that heals your heart doesn't have to be hard. On the contrary, many of my patients who had never enjoyed vigorous exercise find that the exercise they chose for their lifestyle medicine recipe becomes the part of the day they look forward to most and makes them feel energetic rather than tired.

I know what some of you are thinking. Maybe you can't even envision yourself going for a walk around the block, much less going to the gym for thirty minutes. Maybe you even find exercise painful. When your heart is crying out to be healed, exercise is especially intimidating and can indeed be painful, even dangerous. Many of the patients for whom I've helped develop a Precision Personalized Solution, when they first came to see me, were in pain and had to stop and rest while climbing a single flight of stairs. Exercise was the last thing in the world they wanted. But just months later, moderate exercise was as much a part of their enjoyment of improved health as eating good food, drinking clean water, sleeping well, and engaging with their friends and family. And for many of them exercise did not include pursuing sports or going to the gym.

Nighttime

By the time Claire sits down for dinner, the day has delivered a bonfire of inflammatory insults to her system: a hormone burn, a blood sugar spike and then drop, no exercise, and, unbeknownst to her, a food sensitivity. (More on this in a moment!) At home, she pulls the cork on a bottle of wine to accompany dinner and dinner preparation. Between helping the kids with homework, cleaning the kitchen from the morning frenzy, and cooking, Claire downs a couple of glasses of wine before dinner even starts.

Dinner turns out fantastic, and it looks healthy too. The swordfish steak comes off the grill sizzling to perfection, the pasta reminds her of the meals her mom used to make—even though the sauce came from a jar!—and the garlic bread is that perfect combination of soft in the middle and crisp around the edges. To make it "healthier," she replaces the butter in the garlic bread with fat-free margarine. Fat is bad for you, right?

Even the salad looks great, with lettuce, tomato, onion, croutons, and her favorite low-fat salad dressing poured over the top. Since Claire only nibbled at the overcooked broccoli that came with the steak for lunch, this salad is the first serving of vegetables she's had all day. Finally, she serves up her son's favorite dessert: the rest of a sugar-free, whole-wheat carrot cake she made two days earlier.

Unfortunately, although Claire prepared dinner with the healthiest of intentions, the final outcome is more inflammation in her system.

Let's start with that chardonnay. The current recommendation for alcohol consumption for women is one drink per day (and even that small amount is now under question), not the two hefty glasses adding up to more like three units of alcohol that Claire had by the time the dishes were done and the kitchen was cleaned up. Additionally, and unbeknownst to her, she has a genotype, called apolipoprotein E4 allele (ApoE4), that increases the risk of metabolism problems, heart disease, and Alzheimer's—the disease that killed Claire's grandfather. Alcohol has been shown to cause an increase in inflammation associated with an inflammatory protein called C-reactive protein (CRP) in older people with this gene.

The CRP test is part of any thorough blood test, but Claire has never taken a blood test other than the standard cholesterol test at her local health fair and the one recommended by her family physician. There are inexpensive and much more revealing blood tests that can be ordered by your family doctor, but they have yet to catch on in mainstream medicine, even though they provide a great deal of insight into what makes you unique and how to manage your health. (See Chapter 9 for more on CRP and how to ask your doctor for the right blood tests.)

The salad was a good effort, but it was too little too late. In my opinion, one of the biggest reasons for the disease epidemic in America is that we treat vegetables as a side dish—we simply don't eat enough of them while devouring far too much of everything else. That one cup of vegetables per family member in Claire's salad is only about one-third of the amount recommended by the USDA (US Department of Agriculture), which is two and a half cups of vegetables (along with two cups of fruit) per day. Claire is hardly alone, however: according to the Centers for Disease Control and Prevention (CDC), 87 percent of Americans—yes, almost nine out of ten—do not meet fruit and vegetable intake recommendations.

Moreover, I would consider the USDA's recommendation to be misleading, because variety and quality are critical if you want your body to harvest the array of heart-sustaining nutrients available in fruits and vegetables. Eating a salad that is 90 percent pesticide-coated lettuce isn't nearly as nutritious (or tasty) as a salad with a balanced mix of six or seven organic, high-quality, and differently colored vegetables. Vegetables are so important to the proper functioning of our bodies that if you want to make one simple meal-time change to dramatically reduce your risk of vascular disease, lose weight, feel more energetic, and live longer, switch your ratio of carbs and protein to vegetables: eat a pile of veggies, with side orders of carbs and protein. There will be more in Chapter 6 on what veggies to choose and which ones are particularly fantastic for your heart.

Speaking of protein, since fish is full of omega-3, and every health expert trumpets the benefits of eating fish, the tender fillet of swordfish must be good, right? In a world free of pollution, swordfish would be perfectly healthy to eat, but unfortunately that's not the world we live in. Large top predators like swordfish have extremely high levels of toxic compounds, including heavy metals such as mercury. Toxins build up as they move through the food chain, so the larger predators contain the collective toxins from the smaller fish they ate, the prey the smaller fish ate, and so on down the food chain. Yes, the swordfish does contain beneficial omega-3 fatty acids, but the damage caused by the toxins in the meat almost certainly outweighs any advantage gained from the fatty acids. Additionally, if we want to enjoy fish (both in the sea and on our plates) for long into the future, we need to think about the issue of overfishing. Any fish market worth a sardine will recommend fish choices that are both low-mercury and harvested with consideration for sustaining the species.

Soy

Now let's look at some of those juicy ingredients in Claire's salad dressing and the margarine on her garlic bread. The first ingredient in both is soybean oil. It's estimated that 20 percent of the calories in the American diet come from soybeans, most of them in heavily processed derivatives of soy like soybean oil. If you were deficient in omega-6, soybean oil would be a great supplement to balance your fatty acids, but we just learned that we already consume far too much omega-6.

Proponents of soy will tell you that the Japanese, some of the healthiest people in the world, have been eating soy for centuries, and they live longer than we do, so soy must be healthy. However, the problem is the way we eat it. The Japanese eat most of their soy in a less-processed form, like edamame, miso, natto (fermented soybeans) or tofu, and dried soybeans, which are less harmful (read: inflammatory) than soy derivatives. Much of the soy we eat is highly processed and hidden in other foods.

Soy contains a toxic chemical called phytohemaglutinin, which has been blamed for slowing circulation, clotting blood, damaging the nervous system, interfering with digestion, and even causing memory loss. But for every point against soy, there is another one trumpeting soy's health benefits. The plant sterol (sort of like plant cholesterol) in soy has been demonstrated to lower cholesterol in humans—but it can also be found in less controversial foods like nuts, beans, and rice bran.

I prefer to assess soy by the same standard I use to assess many other foods: the less processed the better. I tell my patients that tofu, edamame, miso, and natto are probably good soy sources, but that more heavily processed soy products like soymilk, soybean oil, soy "meats," and soy baby formula should probably be avoided. Also avoid using soy to replace meat in every meal and consuming too many soy-based products for snacks. Using organic, non-GMO tofu, natto, and edamame in some of your meals, however, as well as limited amounts of soy sauce in place of salt, is perfectly healthy.

The Problem with Carbohydrates

What about Claire's whole-wheat pasta, the garlic bread, and the carrot cake? They're all made from a healthy whole grain, right? Before we get into the specifics of how this particular grain affects Claire, let's talk a little more about carbohydrates in general. One problem with carbohydrates, aside from the blood sugar and fat storage factors, is quantity: it's the chips you had after work, the sandwich you had for lunch yesterday, the cereal you had for breakfast the day before, the pizza you had for dinner for two nights in a row, and so on—all the way back to your childhood. Most of us consume far more carbohydrates than our bodies can burn. If you're an athlete, you can handle a higher carbohydrate load than someone with a more sedentary lifestyle, and emerging research suggests that individuals tolerate, and benefit from, carbohydrates very differently. But on average, Americans should cut their carbohydrate consumption in half. We consume about 250 to 300 grams of carbs each day—over half of our total calorie consumption.

And here's the biggest problem with that whole-wheat pasta when it comes to Claire's particular biology: she has an intolerance to gluten, one of the substances in wheat. Scientists have called gluten an "anti-nutrient" because of its damaging potential and distinct lack of benefit to the body. At best, gluten has no impact on the human body, positive or negative; at worst, it's poison. For Claire, gluten is the latter. Her immune system thinks gluten is an invader, so anytime she eats wheat, her body goes into attack mode. Because wheat is in just about every meal she eats, her system is always in attack mode—and therefore always inflamed.

Food Sensitivity

Food sensitivity and the similar food intolerance are among the hottest and most compelling concepts in internal medicine right now, but our understanding of how they work on an individual level is still in its infancy. We've made it over the first big hurdle: recognizing that food sensitivity is a real problem. I'll explain how food sensitivity works in more detail in the next chapter. For the moment, think of it as a low-grade allergic reaction that continues over a long period of time, creating a cycle of inflammation with deleterious consequences for virtually all of the body's systems.

One of the most damaging consequences of Claire's several-times-daily dose of wheat for her entire life has been the degradation of her body's filters—the tightly packed walls of epithelial cells that are critical for keeping stuff where it's supposed to be. Epithelial cells line the blood vessels and intestines, and a specialized kind of epithelial cell makes up the blood-brain barrier, which allows essential nutrients and beneficial cells to pass into the brain while keeping out many of the more damaging substances in the bloodstream.

Over the years, as the epithelial filtering cells of Claire's small intestine became inflamed, the bond between the epithelial cells loosened, allowing incompletely digested nutrients to escape from the intestines into her bloodstream and the intestinal cavity without going through the proper epithelial filter. This in turn compounded the inflammatory response as her body's cleanup crew became over-whelmed with the mess caused by the failure of the epithelial filters. This is the intestinal permeability, or leaky gut syndrome, that I was scolded for speaking of during my residency. While our understand-ing of the process is still developing, we do know it is closely associ-ated with Crohn's disease, ulcerative colitis, and other autoimmune issues. In the brain, the breakdown of the blood-brain barrier may precede Alzheimer's disease.

So even though Claire is eating whole grains, her sensitivity to wheat is moving her heart toward a disease state without her knowl-edge, or her doctor's. As you can see, inflammation sets up a nasty cycle: inflammation begets more inflammation, and food and life-style choices can either increase or decrease inflammation every day. Here's a way of looking at the potential damage from inflammation that should help: There are two kinds of medical conditions in the body—absolute and relative. A broken leg is absolute—you either have a broken leg or you do not. There's no in between. Most chronic dis-eases, on the other hand, including diabetes and other heart diseases, are relative conditions. Sure, a heart attack or stroke is an acute and absolute incident, but scientists have drawn a line in the sand for the conditions that can lead up to these acute incidents: if you fall on one side of the line, you're sick (such as diabetic), and if you're on the other side of the line, you are not.

Understanding the difference between relative and absolute conditions reveals the danger of waiting until diagnosis before treating the disease. Claire may be speeding toward obesity, diabetes, heart attack, or stroke, neither realizing it nor being warned about it, because she has not yet been given a specific diagnosis.

The End of the Inflammatory Day

Claire's story is a compendium of the personal stories that many of my patients tell when they arrive in my clinic. They are *trying*, sometimes desperately, to do the right thing for their health. They aren't eating pizza and cake at every meal, and most of them are managing to keep everything together—including their families, jobs, personal lives, professional lives, hobbies, kids, and friendships—all while suffering from less than optimal health. If parts of Claire's story felt rather close to home for you, you're not alone.

In my practice, inflammation is my greatest enemy (and my patients'). If a patient and I can't reduce the inflammation in her body, it is nearly impossible to stop her painful slide toward dysfunction. If we can reduce her inflammation, however, beautiful things happen: not only are her symptoms of disease reduced, but other inflammation-related issues and her quality of life are improved. Much of the functional medicine protocol you'll find in Part III is designed to reduce inflammation, and the result never ceases to amaze and inspire me with the surprising and wonderful things that happen far from the injury we're trying to treat. Many women I've treated for severe conditions such as heart disease, dementia, diabetes, or fibromyalgia also had joint pain like a sore knee or other problem far from their primary complaint; then they've told me during a follow-up: "I'm feeling much better, and by the way, my knee stopped hurting." If you are serious about pursuing heart health, and implement the plan you will have in mind by the end of this book, be ready to be pleasantly surprised at how your body's trouble spots tend to fade away.

One of the most important messages I have to share with you is a little different from what some of my colleagues are saying. While they describe the quest for a healthier lifestyle with words like "epic" and "dramatic" and "hard," I can say that my patients have shown me that the changes you can make to shift your path from heading toward disease to heading toward vitality are usually not all that significant. Most of my patients have maintained much of their lifestyle while simply identifying and adjusting a few areas that are causing them the most trouble.

For example, how much would Claire have to do to change the dinner described earlier from one that increases inflammation to one that reduces inflammation? Depending on her unique body, probably not very much. In Claire's dinner, just a few small changes would have made a significant difference: using a little butter from grass-fed cows rather than margarine, replacing the sour cream with organic yogurt and the swordfish with wild-caught salmon or another low-mercury fish, increasing the salad portion and the diversity of vegetables in the salad. And considering her wheat sensitivity, Claire would do well to replace the whole-wheat pasta and garlic bread with gluten-free versions.

Your own heart doesn't work that differently from Claire's or most other women's, but how your heart interacts with the environment to which it's subjected make you different from every other woman you know, even those genetically closest to you like your sister or mother. To help you learn the language of your unique body, the following two chapters explore how the key systems of your body work together. Your unique imbalances lie in this relationship—as do your greatest opportunities to heal your heart and live a long and vital life.

Chapter 4

The Functional
Medicine Quartet

Heart, Genes, Brain, and Gut

Now that I've explained inflammation and how it creeps into your daily life in insidious ways, the next step is to share with you the functional medicine anatomy lesson I share with every woman who visits my clinic. I teach them about the interaction of their heart, brain, gut, and genes through the messaging of hormones, the nutrient delivery of the vascular system, and the metabolic process of energy use. Viewing this information through the lens of her own intuition and familiarity with herself, each of these women becomes more knowledgeable about where her imbalances are than I could ever be, even with my double master's degree and four board certifications.

Here we'll examine the four elements of what I call the functional medicine quartet to help you develop a baseline understanding of how the systems of your body work together, pinpoint your own imbalances, and determine a solution that is best for you.

The Heart

By now you know quite a bit about the incredible mechanism of the heart and how it works. But did you know that the human heart not only pumps blood but also plays a role in your personality, energy, and state of mind?

For some time we've been good at operating on and even transplanting the heart, but we're learning that there is more to the heart than just being the body's durable, mechanical pump. Heart transplant patients have found that with their new heart comes a change in personality and behavior. Subconscious memories and feelings are transplanted from one human into another with a transplanted heart, and science has few explanations for how this happens.

Researchers in the late 1970s and early '80s examined hormones produced and released by the heart, including noradrenaline (stress-related), dopamine (makes you feel good), and oxytocin (associated with snuggling, love, and bonding). One result of this research was the inclusion of the heart as one of the body's endocrine glands—part of the hormonal system.

Western culture doesn't look upon heart energy with the same reverence that many other cultures do, but considering phrases like "Put some heart into it" or "I don't have the heart for that," it's clear that we do recognize something emotional about heart energy, even if we don't have a name for it. In Chinese culture, this energy is called *chi*; it's known as *prana* in Tibet and India, which consider it the most powerful of all the body's energy centers. Hawaiians and Polynesians call it *mana*. The Native American Haudenosaunee tribe calls it *orendam*, and the Ituraea pygmies of the African Congo call it *megbe*. Twenty-five years ago, I spent two weeks studying with a 100-year-old Mayan healer in Belize who called it *sastun*; through touch and vibrational energy, he accessed the signature in one's *sastun* to determine which medicine in nature, in the form of healing herbs, was needed. He called it the "signature of nature": the theory that the heart tells you what it needs from nature if you listen in just the right way.

Why Is Mitochondria DNA Different from Our Own DNA?

Scientists speculate that somewhere along the evolutionary journey, mitochondria came from bacteria that made their way into the muscle cells of a primordial animal. Taking up residence, these bacteria then began a mutually beneficial relationship with the animal. The host animal gave the bacteria a home, and the bacteria's energy conversion gave the host animal the most efficient energy-processing method of any living thing. The rest is history.

No matter what you call it, when doctors listen to your heart with a stethoscope, order an MRI or EKG, or even enter your heart through surgical procedures, they learn something about how your heart is functioning physically—but nothing about its emotional health. There is only one person who can assess the emotional health of your heart: *you*.

Along with pumping blood and driving emotion in profound ways, the heart is the control room for your entire body's energy use. No supercomputer could model the incredibly complex endocrine, genetic, and electrical energy patterns your heart generates as it communicates with every one of the 50 trillion or more cells in your body. You may remember from high school biology that the mitochondria in your cells are your cellular power plants. The cells in your heart need much more energy than other cells, and they have far more mitochondria. Each heart cell contains about five thousand mitochondria—more than twice as many as the two thousand mitochondria in a bicep muscle cell. About 5 percent of your body mass consists of mitochondria. The DNA in your mitochondria is different from the DNA in the rest of you, and, ironically, for a society that has given women's hearts short shrift, genetic research suggests that you inherit mitochondria DNA from your mom, not your dad!

It wasn't long ago that the medical community viewed heart disease as an untreatable, irreversible chronic disease, and those who were genetically susceptible to it as doomed. This view was just like mainstream medicine's current view of Alzheimer's disease and diabetes. (Functional medicine is now demonstrating, however, that diabetes and even Alzheimer's can be treated if aggressive, precisely personalized therapies are initiated soon enough.) Starting in the 1970s, Nobel Prize winner Linus Pauling led a few other doctors in championing the cause of cellular health through "orthomolecular medicine"—a fancy term for targeted nutrition. Then, with improved scanning technology that revealed the enormous healing capability of a properly nurtured body and visionary lifestyle medicine therapies like Dr. Ornish's heart disease reversal program, the medical community changed its tune on heart disease: now we see heart disease as something that can be treated, reversed, and prevented. Mechanical failures of the heart's main working parts are extremely rare, and your heart is quite likely to perform perfectly for a lifetime if you give it the essential nutrients and emotional nourishment it needs. And even if you've given your heart a few knocks in the past, the solution I'm sharing with you in this book will enable you to harness its incredible ability to heal, grow stronger, and power you throughout a future free of disease.

We now know that nutrition, lifestyle, diet, and exercise are the keys to keeping a person with a genetic susceptibility to heart disease from ever getting it. We also have observed that a person without a genetic susceptibility to heart disease can nevertheless, through poor nutrition and lifestyle choices, become overweight, diabetic, and hypertensive (high blood pressure), develop dangerous cholesterol imbalances, and eventually suffer an early death from heart disease. We'll talk momentarily about how the environment influences our genes, but the breakthrough understanding in genetics in recent years is that you have a choice: you can turn on your bad genes through bad lifestyle choices, or you can turn on your good genes that protect you by making heart-smart choices.

The Genes

Your genes are your potential, not your destiny . . . Your genes are your potential, not your destiny . . . Your genes are your potential, not your destiny. . . . Keep this mantra in mind as you read the rest of *Heart Solution for Women*. Even better, keep it in mind for the rest of your life. Regardless of your family history or current risk for heart disease, diabetes, obesity, high blood pressure, or dangerous cholesterol levels, you can change your genetic potential for the better. The idea that we can manipulate the way our cells interact with our genes may be mind-blowing, but it is a key part of your solution.

The Human Genome Project, a collaborative international research project to map all the genes of the human genome (genetic material), revealed that many of biology's most cherished tenets about genetic determinism to be part of the 50 percent we had wrong when I was in medical school. How your environment affects your health and your genes is turning out to be much more important than the genes you inherited from your ancestors. Researchers have called the idea that genetic destiny rules our health a "Darwinian hangover." A study of 1.5 million deaths from heart disease and cancer revealed that only 16 percent were caused by genetic factors. Single-gene disorders are even rarer, affecting less than 2 percent of the population.

The genetics we were taught in high school—we're machines controlled by fixed aspects of our DNA—is now giving way to an understanding that our genes and our lifestyle choices are powerful cocreators of our lives and that we have much more control over our destinies than we ever imagined. The term for this new understanding is "epigenetics." The prefix epi- means *above, besides*, or *in addition to*. For our purposes, epigenetics explains how it isn't so much the genes you were born with that determine whether you'll live a long and vital life or die young from disease, but the factors *besides* the DNA you were born with that influence how your genes react to your environment throughout your life. And in a world where your lifestyle choices dramatically influence the environment in which your cells are bathed, your conscious decisions very much drive your epigenetic potential—good and bad.

The new science of epigenetics has provided the missing link in our quest to prevent heart disease as well as other chronic diseases. Epigenetics is proving that environment can overcome the predetermination your genes patterned—for better or worse. Epigenetics is showing that what happens to your health as you age is not chiseled in stone by your DNA but instead is the result of a fluid, changing interaction between the environment and your genetics. Your genes pick the instrument, but it's your environment and lifestyle choices that play the music.

Initially, researchers believed that to control the many complex processes involved in the workings of a human body, the Human Genome Project would have to discover about 120,000 genes. But then, when the human genome was mapped out, it turned out that we only have about 22,000 genes. Somehow 80 percent of our expected genetic matter turned up missing! Researchers looked at other organisms and found that the size of an organism's genome doesn't correlate to the organism's complexity. Mice have 1,000 more genes than humans, fruit flies have almost as many, and amphibians have thirty times more. Do the more than 30,000 genes of a merlot grape—even a grape destined for the glories of wine—make it more complex than a human? These mind-blowing discoveries changed everything about our perception of genetic destiny and begged the question: If DNA is everything, how do we explain the vibrant and complex variation and capabilities in humans versus the seemingly simple life of a frog?

Our 22,000 genes are made up of building blocks called nucleotides, which are arranged in pairs. There are 3 billion nucleotides in the human genome. (Now we're getting somewhere in explaining human complexity and variation!) One particular part of DNA, single nucleotide polymorphisms (which has such a tongue twister of a name that they are referred to as SNPs, pronounced "snips") have been compared to sticky notes placed on your DNA by your environment and your experiences. This process is called epigenetic expression—the language of how your genes react to your environment.

Scientists estimate that there are over 10 million SNP variations. With the discovery of SNPs and epigenetic expression, the significance of lifestyle choices, and today's most exciting avenue for prevention and treatment of chronic disease, was revealed.

The old set-in-stone concept of genetics failed to recognize the significance of epigenetic expression, which works like this: Your DNA is not changed by environmental factors, but the environment does influence how your SNPs respond. Many researchers also now believe that a cell's membrane—which is only seven millionths of a millimeter thick—controls how its genes express themselves by turning them on and off, depending on the cell's environment. When placed in a nutrient-rich environment, the cell turns on the growth gene and divides and grows new tissue. When placed in a toxic or stressful environment, the cell's membrane closes its doors, circles the wagons, and turns on its inflammatory genes in an attempt to keep out anything harmful.

At first glance, this binary view of epigenetics appears overly simplistic, but it makes perfect sense if we remember that a wild animal is usually in one of two modes: either thriving or fighting for its life. An animal is either sleeping, eating, and reproducing (thriving) or trying not to starve, avoiding being eaten, and healing, if necessary, from narrow escapes (fighting). It follows that the animal's cells would respond to these two basic modes.

The founder of the Institute for Functional Medicine, Dr. Jeffrey Bland, explains it this way in his excellent book *The Disease Delusion*: "There are no superior genes, there are only superior diet, lifestyle and environment, and we all have an equal genetic opportunity to create them for ourselves." Of course, there are genetic mutations that can spell a death sentence or disease for some individuals, but these are exceedingly rare compared to the dance of genes and the environment, which affects us all equally.

Let's say you have a pattern of SNPs that are sensitive to messaging triggered by excessive sugar in the cell's environment. When the cell is then repeatedly exposed to the inflammatory messaging of excessive sugar, these SNPs are turned on and eventually you are diagnosed with type 2 diabetes, a "genetic" disease. Conversely, if you don't expose those same SNPs to an environment with too much sugar, they'll never be turned on and you won't be diagnosed with diabetes.

Say you don't cut back on sugar soon enough. Well, here's the silver lining: certain nutrients have been shown to turn off, or soothe, SNPs. This soothing of the SNPs is called methylation. When SNPs are methylated, they are less likely to be activated by environmental influences. In other words, methylation can prevent "bad" genes from being turned on as easily. (I know what you're thinking—hang tight, I'll share these nutrients with you soon.) Therefore—and this might be the most important message in this book—even if you are predisposed to a certain disease, nutrients found in food and nutritional supplements can prevent your chronic disease–causing SNPs patterns from being turned on, and if they are turned on, these nutrients can turn them off.

This is wild, right? But as we'd say in Wyoming, hang on to your hat, it gets wilder. When you reproduce, most of your epigenetic markers are erased, granting your offspring a relatively clean slate. However, cutting-edge research in epigenetics has shown that, in a process called transgenerational epigenetic inheritance, some SNPs "sticky notes" make it through the process of reproduction and can pass from parent to child and even on to grandchildren, sometimes skipping a generation. This is a shocking concept: not only can you influence your genes through your choices and lifestyle, but your parents' and grandparents' lifestyle and nutrition choices turned on SNPs of your DNA that contribute to the person you are today. And your choices, in turn, will influence your children's and grandchildren's epigenetic inheritance.

These discoveries are only just beginning to influence the front lines of the practice of medicine. Many doctors will still tell you that your chances of having a heart attack are primarily determined by your DNA and whether or not your parents died of a heart attack— and they're half-right. Your genes do influence your chances of getting heart disease, but not the way we learned in school. We used to think our genes were predetermined and we had no influence over them.

We were told it was just the luck of the genetic draw as to whether or not we would get the disease. Probably the best medical news of our generation is that this just ain't so.

Consider these two examples of epigenetics: the Pima Indians and the Agouti mice.

The Pima Indians of Arizona typically marry other Pima, so they have proven to be an incredible resource for epigenetic research. Traditionally, diabetes and obesity were unheard of in the Pima tribe, but today 50 percent of Pimas are diabetic, and 95 percent of those who are diabetic are overweight. The DNA of the Pima is the same as it was 100 years ago, but the epigenetic expression has changed in response to their environment. The theory is that over thousands of years the Pima developed what scientists call a "thrifty" gene in response to living in an environment with alternating periods of feast and famine. The thrifty gene allowed them to store nutrients in their bodies during times of plenty to better endure the times of famine. Now, with the environmental influence of famine removed entirely, replaced by the environmental influence of a Western diet and lifestyle, that same thrifty marker makes the Pima extraordinarily susceptible to diabetes and obesity. Did their genes change in 100 years? Not at all! But the information bathed over those thrifty genes changed, and it made the Pima Indians genetically predisposed to diabetes and obesity, even though their ancestors with the same DNA were not.

On the bright side of epigenetics and the promise of methylation is the breakthrough study on the effects of methylation in Agouti mice and the influence of nutrition on diseases with a genetic component. The Agouti mice were bred to be diabetic and obese with an increased risk for cancer, and they also had characteristic yellow coats. With no methylation treatment, the offspring of the Agouti mice were also diabetic, obese, cancer-prone, and yellow. But when the mothers were treated with an advanced methylation therapy (including methylated B12, methyl folate, and zinc, all elements of the Precision, Personalized Solution), the offspring were born absolutely healthy, free of diabetes, normal weight, and without increased cancer risk. They even had ordinary brown coats—the methylation had prevented not only the diseases but even the hair color of the mothers from being passed on to their offspring.

Methylation is a key element in the practice of functional medicine, and I include it in the majority of my patients' solutions. It isn't complex and can be done through nutritional supplementation, including methylated B12, found in just about every health food store. In Chapter 8, I'll give you guidelines for methylation supplements, but here the next step is to consider how the brain interacts with both the heart and genes.

The Brain

There may be no part of the body steeped in urban myth more than the brain. We've long been told that we use only 10 percent of our brains, but it turns out that we use 100 percent. We've been told that we're either left brain– or right brain–dominant, but MRI scans have revealed that while certain functions are centered in specific parts of our brains, neither side is dominant over the other. It turns out that the creative person isn't right brain–dominant and the detail-oriented person isn't left brain–dominant. We've been told that playing classical music for fetuses makes them smarter, that subliminal messages hidden in music and movies affect our decision-making, and that brain injuries cannot heal. These theories of the brain have been largely proven incorrect but are still deeply entrenched in our society.

Then there are the facts about the brain that are far less well known but should be making headline news. For example, a mother can boost her child's IQ by more than three and a half points by consuming omega-3 during pregnancy. Heavy marijuana consumption as a teenager can reduce IQ by nearly ten points. Imperceptible strokes (microinfarcts) due to reduced vascular function limit oxygen to the brain and can result in dementia. (The good news is that improved heart function reduces dementia risk.) The list goes on. I'd go so far as to say that most of us would be better off forgetting everything we've learned about the brain and replacing it with all new information so that we can take better care of that mysterious machine between our ears.

Your brain contains about 86 billion neurons connected by synapses that are fed nutrients through 100,000 miles of capillaries—more blood vessels than the rest of your body combined. One of the most misunderstood brain features is the specialized capillary structure of the blood-brain barrier, that border patrol between your body and brain that keeps many blood-borne pathogens and other undesirables from getting into your brain while letting nutrient-rich blood pass freely. The blood-brain barrier is an endless challenge for pharmacologists, as many medications cannot penetrate the barrier. Some immune cells are allowed past the barrier and others are not. Some vitamins pass the barrier and others do not. Sneaky diseases like HIV and herpes disguise themselves to slip past, and many inflammatory molecules can also cross the blood-brain barrier.

I was taught in medical school that the ills of the brain were unique to the brain, and that the ills of the body were largely kept out of the brain. To this day, the status quo approach to the prevention and treatment of disease is limited by this old perception, reinforced by misunderstandings of the blood-brain barrier, that the brain is somehow separate from the rest of the body. It turns out that many things, including chronic inflammation, affect both the body and brain. For our purposes here, we can't develop a solution to save your heart without considering the health of your brain.

More than ever before, we're learning that a properly functioning brain and nervous system relies on a properly functioning heart and cardiovascular system. Terms like "synaptic plasticity" are used to describe the strengthening or weakening of neuron connections, while arterial flexibility describes the health of the arterial wall. Consider the similar physical manifestations of Alzheimer's and heart disease. In victims of cardiovascular disease, biopsies show plaques, mostly made of cholesterol, lining the arteries. In biopsies of Alzheimer's victims, the brain is choked with two visually dramatic features: plaques of beta-amyloid proteins surrounding the synapses and nerve fibers, which apparently are choked by tau proteins shaped into chaotic tangles. In heart disease, the decline of arterial function limits the delivery of oxygen and other nutrients to needy organs and tissues. In Alzheimer's, the decline of neural pathways limits the delivery of information and nutrients, so the nerve cells eventually die. Many of the risk factors for Alzheimer's are also risk factors for heart disease. A close relative of Alzheimer's, vascular dementia, is caused by reduced blood flow to the brain due to heart issues. In fact, there are so many similarities between heart disease and Alzheimer's that some researchers are now calling Alzheimer's type 3 diabetes.

Heart disease is caused by chronic inflammation in the vasculature of the heart and arteries, and Alzheimer's is caused by chronic inflammation in the vasculature of the brain. Diabetes, typically viewed as a cardiovascular disease, can damage nerve fibers so badly that it eventually causes nerve death. The medical establishment would do well to embrace this categorization of Alzheimer's as a vascular disease and type 3 diabetes. The simple change of nomenclature could change the way we look at the disease and open doors for powerful collaboration between medical specialties. Sure, the symptoms of heart disease, diabetes, and Alzheimer's are very different, but when it comes to prevention and healing, the three are almost identical. This is why, in my practice, I view heart disease and Alzheimer's, from a curative perspective, *as the same thing.* This is also why your own Precision, Personalized Solution will dramatically reduce not only your heart disease risk but also your Alzheimer's risk.

I'm not alone in this view—other doctors and researchers also advocate the reclassification of Alzheimer's from a disease isolated to the brain to a disease of the entire body that manifests itself in the brain. Dr. Mark Hyman, my friend and colleague in functional medicine, shares my view of Alzheimer's as a vascular disease that can be prevented and even treated in its early stages. As he explains in his blog:

> Just like we once thought that heart disease and artery-clogging plaques couldn't be reversed (and now have proof that this does happen), I believe dementia can be reversed (if caught

early enough) by attending to all the factors that affect brain function—diet, exercise, stress, nutritional deficiencies, toxins, hormonal imbalances, inflammation, and more.

The revelations of the connection between brain and heart health have shattered the traditional view that the brain's health is somehow separate from that of the rest of the body. We now know that what's good for the heart is also good for the brain—and that what damages the heart also damages the brain. This is why, in my observation, individuals who commit themselves to decision-making and lifestyle therapies that support a healthy heart often heal from depression, improve mental energy and focus, and regain much of their youthful countenance.

But none of this can happen without considering the gut—the final instrument of the quartet. Discussion about disease has traditionally pushed the gut to the sidelines to focus on the high-profile players—the heart, the brain, and genetics. But with the recent revelations about the importance of the microbiome (the trillions of bacterial cells living in the gut) and the potential damage caused by the immune system, it turns out that the gut is center stage.

The Gut

Of the four instruments of the functional medicine quartet, *the gut provides us with the greatest opportunity to heal.* For this reason, the gut is the target of the majority of the therapies I use in my clinic and will teach you in this book. The gut has been called the second brain. The mighty web of neurons lining and surrounding the intestines is in constant communication with the heart and brain, and the majority of the body's powerful immune response is initiated in the gut.

The connection between the gut and the brain is called the vagus nerve. It functions as the super-highway of communication between your brain and gut. The vagus nerve is known as the "wandering nerve" as it weaves its way down from the brain stem to the lower abdomen, interacting with most organs along the way, including the heart. There are chemical messengers going down the vagus nerve from the brain to the gut, yet far more messages travel upwards, from the gut to the brain.

So closely are the heart, brain, and gut tied together that researchers have theorized that the vagus nerve is a mediator for the relationship between inflammation, heart disease, depression, and metabolic syndrome (a dangerous combination of high blood sugar, concerning cholesterol levels, high blood pressure, and excess body fat around the waist). Fifteen years ago, therapists experimented with a vagus nerve electrical stimulation device to treat patients with depression and mood disorders. In my experience, however, a far more effective stimulation for the vagus nerve is proper nutrition—and sure enough, improved nutrition results in improved mood.

The crucial thing to know about the gut is that one woman's medicine is another woman's poison. How your particular body handles the stuff you eat is determined by three primary factors: first, what kind of nutrients you consume and then actually absorb; second, how your gut responds to the information in the nutrients; and third, the condition of your small intestine.

Think of your gut as your nutrient post office. It's where the mess of information in the food you eat is organized to be delivered. When the absorbing cells are working effectively, the nutrients are transformed to usable energy or the building blocks your body needs. When the absorbing cells are not working optimally, nutrients are not all absorbed; instead of being transported through the appropriate channels for your body to use, some nutrients either pass through your gut unused or leak between the cells. Caused by the permeability of the intestine, this is leaky gut syndrome, and its discovery completely shifted how we view women's health and the significance of the symptoms of intestinal discomfort so many women frequently describe.

The next time you are hanging out with your girlfriends, ask how many of them have digestive issues. Most of them will raise their hands. Then ask them how many have told their doctors about these issues. Hands still up. Then ask how many were told to ignore it, since most women have digestive problems. Hands still up. Far too many of my female patients have digestive issues and have been told it's "normal" or just to ignore it. I have heard this not only from my patients but also from my own doctor when I was having digestive issues. (I'll tell you my gut story soon.) I am passionate about your heart, which means I care about your gut.

Way back during my residency at Banner University Medical Center in Phoenix, I learned just how controversial this leaky gut concept really was. Walking through the intensive care unit, I was talking with one of the junior residents about the concept of leaky gut when I was stopped by an attending physician, one of the almighty gods of medicine who teaches the underling residents and interns. He said, with the full power of his authority, "Never let those words leave your lips again in my hospital."

I asked him, as meekly as I could, "May I use the term 'intestinal permeability'?"

He thought for a moment. It seemed to me that he obviously didn't know what it was, no matter what term was used. Then he said, "It's still wrong, but acceptable."

Both mainstream medicine and people suffering from the condition remain reluctant to fully embrace leaky gut as a real condition. Most people by now have heard of leaky gut from the internet or from a friend. The most common story goes something like this (and chances are good that one of your female friends could tell you almost this exact story): A woman goes to the doctor for intestinal issues after dealing with gut issues for as long as she can remember: her belly is bloated and painful, and she's in constant discomfort from variable and unpredictable bowel patterns. The doctor tells her: "You have irritable bowel syndrome. You'll just have to learn to live with it. Most women have digestive issues." (You don't want to be told you have a "syndrome," because in medicine that often means your doctor has no idea how to help you.)

With the increased understanding of gut function that has emerged in the last twenty years, I can say with confidence that my attending physician that day was wrong on all counts. Autoimmune disease, which is closely related to permeability of the intestines, has been described by researchers as a pandemic far more commonly found in women than men—ten times more common! Don't believe it's a pandemic? Autoimmune disease is one of the top ten causes of death in female children and women of all ages, affecting more than 23 million Americans. By comparison, cancer affects 13 million Americans.

The anecdotal evidence from my clinic supports the significance of intestinal permeability and autoimmune disease as medical problems as significant as anything the human race has yet faced. I find that nine out of ten women who see me have digestive issues but don't bring them up until I do a complete review of all their systems. Usually what happens is that when we talk about their gut, they downplay the dysfunction because they've been told it's okay and they should try to ignore it. Once their digestive issues are out in the open, we then put together a solution that almost always involves healing their intestines. The point is, no matter what your doctor may have told you, intestinal dysfunction is not okay and you should not ignore it!

The gut is the commander of the body—the most important source of nutritional absorption and detoxification as well as the largest source of mood-stabilizing serotonin. People take antidepressants to balance their serotonin, but it may actually be most effectively balanced by getting rid of the belly bloat and constant discomfort associated with leaky gut. There's a good chance that you'll never need antidepressant medication if you restore the serotonin balance of your gut.

Sounds good, right? But just how do we do this?

One Cell Thick

The first step is understanding leaky gut. Here is how I explain it to my patients: You essentially have a tube running through you, starting at the mouth and ending at the bum. This tube serves as a pipeline for the external environment running through the core of your internal environment.

We tend to think that when we eat something, we magically transform it into something useful and it becomes part of us. This is simply not the case. If we eat a toxin, it remains a toxin. If we eat something we're allergic to, our immune system responds with inflammation. If we accidentally swallow a small rock, it passes through us and emerges just as it went in—as a rock.

The significance of the interaction between the internal environment of the gut and the external environment passing through it was elucidated only recently. The food you eat goes to your stomach, where the acid mushes it up into essentially pudding. Then the lion's share of the action between the internal and external environments takes place in the 26 feet of small intestine, which has a surface area equivalent to a doubles tennis court. The small intestine allows you to absorb the good parts (and many of the bad parts) of the foods you eat. Guess how robust that interface is? The epithelial layer of that doubles tennis court is only one cell thick, and those epithelial cells renew every three days. In other words, the layer separating the outer environment contained in the tube from the robust immune system surrounding your small intestine is vanishingly thin.

The cells of the epithelial layer are connected by proteins that make up a special processing system called the zonulin bridge. Zonulin is a chemical that processes food into a form that is ready for the bloodstream and allows it to pass the border patrol of the immune system and go on to the liver for dissemination as nutrition. If the zonulin bridge fails, food is not processed optimally and gets into the bloodstream without approval by the immune system. This angers the immune system, which then calls in the cytokines, its inflammatory friends. Cytokines are like a chemical Paul Revere that sounds the alarm to alert the defense. The cytokine alarm initiates the antibody defense of the immune system, which then attacks the food particles as if they were parasites. As a result, not only does your inflammation increase, but you lose the nutritional benefit of the food because your body is treating it like an invader rather than a nutrient.

What can make the zonulin bridge fail and give you leaky gut and the ensuing autoimmune disorder? Parasites and really bad viruses and bacteria can do this, and so can heavy metals, smoking, emotional stress, and drugs. (I know, that sounds like the recipe for a great concert, but you wouldn't want it in your belly every day of your life!) Antibiotics can cause leaky gut. Anti-inflammatories can cause leaky gut—one dose of ibuprofen can cause leaky gut in sensitive individuals. Even breast implants can cause leaky gut, because of the immune reaction to the sudden appearance of two foreign objects in the body.

So the antibiotics you took for that urinary tract infection may start this whole damaging process of leaky gut and drive the body into a highly inflamed state. In my opinion, it is hugely irresponsible for doctors to prescribe antibiotics without an accompanying prescription for probiotic and prebiotic supplements and nutritional support to help the microbiome recover from the inevitable and significant damage caused by antibiotics.

Revealing one of those many seemingly contradictory conclusions that can be drawn from medical research, however, a special kind of antibiotic can also improve symptoms of leaky gut, irritable bowel syndrome, and some autoimmune bowel disorders because of its impact on the destructive bacteria living in our intestines. If the antibiotics kill bacteria that are damaging digestive function (which bacteria *sometimes* do), the immune response will probably decrease and the symptoms of intestinal permeability will improve. However, if the antibiotics kill bacteria that are beneficial to digestive function (which antibiotics *always* do), the immune response will almost surely increase and the symptoms of inflammation will worsen.

We have evolved with the bacteria of our guts for millions of years, and every one of us needs bacteria to digest food and, to put it bluntly, live. These bacteria are the microbiome, the little bacterial hitchhikers that live inside us in numbers equal to the number of human cells. (Some researchers have estimated the number of bacterial cells to be far higher, but counting cells is difficult; the most recent evidence suggests that the bacterial count in the body is on the same order of magnitude as the human cell count.) The microbiome is proving to be instrumental in the function of virtually every system in the body.

Taking antibiotics profoundly changes your microbiome, to the point that your microbiome will never be exactly the same afterwards. Antibiotics are powerful medicine that, in my opinion, should be used far less frequently and should always be accompanied by probiotic and prebiotic therapies to bolster the microbiome. The next time your doctor prescribes an antibiotic, ask first if you really need it, and if so, ask for prebiotic, probiotic, and food recommendations to go along with it. (See Chapter 9 for more questions to ask your doctor when they want to prescribe drugs.)

The other drugs that are notorious for damaging the intestinal filters and increasing immune response are the anti-inflammatory meds we take for sore knees and the like. Yes, the common perspective is that ibuprofen, the other NSAIDs (nonsteroidal anti-inflammatory drugs), and similar medications are totally safe, but they're not safe for everyone. They may trigger the Paul Revere cytokine alarm that leads to the uncomfortable symptoms of leaky gut and irritable bowel syndrome and ignites the forest fire of inflammation in the body known as autoimmune disease. Really? One round of antibiotics, taking ibuprofen for a week, or getting breast implants could trigger autoimmune disease? The answer is a resounding YES!

No matter the cause, when the intestines become permeable, a veritable mosh pit of immune cells, food particles, inflammatory hormones, and partially digested nutrients enter the bloodstream. What was supposed to be food cannot be used as nutrition but is now a food protein with an immune protein attached to it. When this happens in a person who is genetically predisposed to joint problems, this protein sandwich becomes an invader and attaches to the person's joints. Then the part of the immune system that does surveillance, floating around the body looking for troublemakers, sees this food particle or antibody complex on the joint tissue and says, "You're not supposed to be there, so I am going to call the forces and attack you." This overreaction against the joint tissue leads to

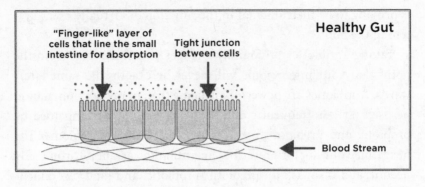

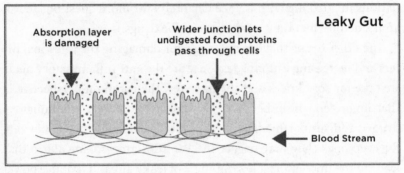

the damage we call rheumatoid arthritis. If you are genetically predisposed to skin issues the immune attack could cause lupus or psoriasis. If you are genetically set up for digestive disease, the immune attack could cause Crohn's disease or ulcerative colitis. And if you are genetically vulnerable to damage in the lining of the blood vessels of the heart, then you end up with a cholesterol plaque that ruptures in a heart attack. Just a little further up, if you are genetically predisposed to brain issues, the immune attack could cause Alzheimer's, Parkinson's disease, or multiple sclerosis.

As you can see, leaky gut is not only absolutely real but is now suspected as a culprit behind a vast range of disease development. But now for the good news. You can fix leaky gut on your own. In Part III, you will learn how to diagnose leaky gut on your own and repair it without a doctor's help. In fact, you're likely to do a better job of it, since many doctors haven't heard of leaky gut, don't understand it, and don't know how to heal it.

Food Sensitivities

In my observation, one of the primary fuels for inflammation and leaky gut is food sensitivity. Every day patients arrive at my clinic saying, "I want that food allergy test that fixed my sister [or brother, or neighbor, etc.]." First of all, it's not a food "allergy" test—it's a food sensitivity and/or intolerance test. What is the difference? A food intolerance is a more dramatic and acute reaction than a food sensitivity, but for the purpose of reducing inflammation by customizing your food choices to best fit your unique biology, we can use the terms interchangeably.

Food allergies are what afflicts the kid in school who eats peanuts and whose face swells up ten minutes later so she has to be taken to the emergency room. This is an immediate histamine reaction from the immune defense system called immunoglobulin E (IgE), and it's the same histamine type of reaction caused by airborne allergens when a cloud of dust (or pollen or mold or dog/cat dander) immediately causes watery eyes and sneezing. We rarely test for food allergies in adults because they learned years earlier what foods give them a histamine response.

While histamine response causes an immediate allergic reaction, food sensitivities caused by the IgG and IgA defense may not produce noticeable symptoms until twenty-four to forty-eight hours later; symptoms can also be more subtle and cumulative, making food sensitivities much more difficult to pinpoint. To make food sensitivity even more confusing, only one in ten food sensitivity symptoms are digestive. That night you slept horribly? That may have been a symptom of sensitivity to the food you ate two days earlier. That Tuesday you had sore joints after some light exercise on Monday? Could have been due to your wheat binge over the weekend.

This delay in food sensitivity reaction is one reason why it is so hard for people to connect the dots. Naturopathic doctors have told their patients for decades about the inflammatory nightshade foods—tomatoes, eggplant, peppers, potatoes, and even those Goji berries full of antioxidants. You may have an inflammatory reaction to nightshades—or they

Healing Leaky Gut Heals Multiple Sclerosis

The most powerful story I've heard about leaky gut is a research series on patients with multiple sclerosis (MS), a devastating disease that robs its victims of strength and nervous system control. They usually end up in a wheelchair—or worse. All ten patients in this clinic study had neurologist-confirmed MS, which is diagnosed with a brain MRI showing a classic "plaque" pattern, spinal fluid with a specific type of protein in it, and the characteristic nervous system and muscular deficiencies.

These ten people fit the medical criteria for MS perfectly, and all were on the medications thought to help MS. None of them got better. Then a functional medicine doctor, noticing that they all had a history of irritable bowel, theorized that the MS was the result of leaky gut causing an autoimmune attack on the brain tissue. The neurologist was very skeptical, but then all ten patients were found to have high antibodies to wheat, including gliadin and gluten, and severe leaky gut based on zonulin markers in the blood showing the breakdown of the protective barrier and activation of the immune system. The ten study participants stopped eating wheat/gluten and followed a protocol designed to heal leaky gut.

Guess what happened? All ten MS patients healed: their muscle function was restored to the point that even the worst afflicted got out of their wheelchairs, and all of them became symptom-free within six months. At that point, they no longer had any medical sign of MS—except that the brain lesions visible with MRI never went away, making their scans look like those of a person with MS.

may treat you wonderfully! As with everything I will teach you about nutrition, our goal is to figure out what foods you should consume or avoid, not what foods have worked for someone else or what works for the average person.

Last year I saw a friend of mine at an international congress. Three years earlier, she had been wheelchair-bound because of MS. When I went to run on the treadmill the second morning of the conference, she was on the treadmill next to me jogging. We had a great conversation about how she healed her leaky gut and healed her MS, even though her doctors thought she was crazy to try and told her it would never work. She still has the MS lesions in her brain, but her body now works.

Think about it: healing leaky gut healed ten out of ten people who had been diagnosed with MS, as well as my friend! The current theory of most autoimmune disease is that leaky gut is a driving force of the illness, and maybe even the root cause. This matters most to you—women are twelve times more likely to have autoimmune disease than men, and 75 percent of people with autoimmune disease are women! What's more, a woman with one autoimmune disease is ten times more likely to develop a second autoimmune disease. Fire breeds fire. Let's put out the fire together.

I see similar improvements every week in my clinic, not only with MS but with conditions like neuropathy, Hashimoto's thyroiditis, colitis, fibromyalgia, chronic fatigue—and heart disease. You have to put out the gut fire to put out the heart and brain fires, and one of the best ways to start is to stop pouring fuel on the gut fire—in the form of foods that trigger your body's immune response.

Your digestive tract has two departments of defense: the IgA system lining the digestive tract and serving as your first barrier to foods your body may not like, and the IgG system in the bloodstream, which provides long-term surveillance and protection. Certain foods can cause a reaction at the IgA mucosal (lining) barrier and then activate the long-term IgG antibodies to keep those foods from causing trouble. Food sensitivities can overactivate this system, leading to autoimmune disease. So a critical part of your solution is to determine which foods activate your defensive system. If you're sensitive to foods you eat every day, or even just weekly or monthly, it is very difficult to heal because the inflammation caused by that sensitivity is always there. It can manifest in a number of ways: as chronic skin issues like eczema or acne, as poor sleep, as nonoptimal mood if it affects the serotonin in your gut, as vague joint pain and fatigue (fibromyalgia), or even as brain fog, poor concentration, or ADD. For women, food sensitivity is notorious for causing thyroid, adrenal, and hormone disruption—all of which eventually damage the heart.

So, now it's time to tell you my own food sensitivity and leaky gut story as promised. I grew up with digestive dysfunction and endured crampy stomach pain and four to six bowel movements every day. My family thought it was funny that I went to the bathroom right after every meal and that they had to make sure it was not already in use by one of the other six kids. I played soccer and could not eat on game day or I would spend halftime in the bathroom and miss part of the second half. Many of the athletes I see in my clinic have this issue, commonly referred to as "runner's gut." Growing up, I was told my problem was lactose intolerance, so I stopped drinking milk and eating cheese for a year. No improvement. I was tested, poked, prodded, and scoped. No answers. At one point I was told by a psychiatrist friend of the family that it was "in my head." Eventually, my doctor prescribed Zelnorm, a medication for irritable bowel syndrome. Luckily for me, before I could get my prescription filled the medicine was pulled from the market owing to the unpleasant side effect of death through bleeding of the bowels.

I found my solution after I had my blood tested for food sensitivities and used the results to change my food choices and heal my leaky gut. Now I have healthy digestion, daily bowel movements, and no pain. The only side effects of paying attention to my food sensitivities have been better sleep, no more pain in the knee I had surgery on in high school, and clearer focus.

The chart reproduced on pages 110–111 is my own food sensitivity panel. Before I was tested for food sensitivities, I ate an egg nearly every day, thinking it was a great protein source for an athlete. I ate bananas every day like a monkey because I'd heard that, with all the long-distance running during training and games, soccer players need potassium. I tried to go vegan by eating legumes and beans. Also, I loved bread. As you can see from my chart, despite my good intentions, I was poisoning myself a little every day.

I have a strong reaction to egg white as well as the casein protein and whey in dairy products, but react less to goat's milk. I react to many kinds of beans, chocolate, sesame, and yeast. This is information I use every day now in making food choices—and I feel better because of it. Food sensitivity and the direct measurement cholesterol tests are the most helpful diagnostic tools to support lifestyle medicine and the most common blood tests I do in my clinic.

Although food sensitivity tests open a revealing window to the culprits behind many health issues, they are not 100 percent accurate, they may be misleading due to false positives, and eliminating some foods you're sensitive to can cause poor nutrition. So even if you get this blood test, it is important to conduct your own experiment to make sure that you're really reacting to the foods suggested by the blood test and also that you're getting plenty of proper nutrition by replacing foods you cut from your diet with others that provide similar nutrients.

This is why, in my world of functional medicine, we don't rely on a single test to determine treatment, and we don't treat just one body part. The Precision, Personalized Solution involves nutrition and lifestyle choices that nurture, monitor, and tune all four instruments in the functional medicine quartet: the heart, the brain, the gut, and the epigenetic response.

With food sensitivities, it's not that your immune system is going out of control to the point of causing a full-blown allergic reaction, but

96 Food IgG Panel

DAIRY				Bar (500–1500)
Casein	1292	High	1	▇▇▇▇▇▇▇▇
Cheddar Cheese	708	Moderate	2	▇▇▇
Cottage Cheese	1180	High	3	▇▇▇▇▇▇▇
Cow's Milk	1356	High	4	▇▇▇▇▇▇▇▇
Goat's Milk	614	Moderate	5	▇
Mozzarella Cheese	932	High	6	▇▇▇▇▇
Whey	1402	High	7	▇▇▇▇▇▇▇▇▇
Yogurt	997	High	8	▇▇▇▇▇

MEAT/FOWL				
Beef	257	No Reaction	9	
Chicken	618	Moderate	10	▇
Duck	192	No Reaction	11	
Egg White	1608	Very High	12	▇▇▇▇▇▇▇▇▇▇
Egg Yolk	584	Moderate	13	▇
Lamb	201	No Reaction	14	
Pork	343	Very Low	15	
Turkey	273	Very Low	16	

SEAFOOD				
Clam	539	Moderate	17	▇
Cod	709	Moderate	18	▇▇
Crab	385	Low	19	
Halibut	334	Very Low	20	
Lobster	297	Very Low	22	
Oyster	630	Moderate	22	▇
Salmon	238	No Reaction	23	
Scallop	208	No Reaction	24	
Shrimp	244	No Reaction	25	
Sole	221	No Reaction	26	
Yellowfin Tuna	168	No Reaction	27	

VEGETABLES				
Asparagus	261	No Reaction	28	
Avocado	231	No Reaction	29	
Beet	297	Very Low	30	
Broccoli	148	No Reaction	31	
Cabbage	530	Low	32	▇
Carrot	470	Low	33	
Cauliflower	352	Very Low	34	
Celery	589	Moderate	35	▇
Cucumber	285	Very Low	36	
Garlic	293	Very Low	37	
Green Pepper	255	No Reaction	38	
Lettuce	296	Very Low	39	
Mushroom	259	No Reaction	40	
Olive	329	Very Low	41	
Onion	186	No Reaction	42	
Potato	170	No Reaction	43	
Pumpkin	197	No Reaction	44	
Radish	235	No Reaction	45	
Spinach	328	Very Low	46	
Tomato	178	No Reaction	47	
Zucchini Squash	225	No Reaction	48	

FRUIT			
Apple	420	Low	49
Apricot	313	Very Low	50
Banana	1061	High	51
Blueberry	429	Low	52
Cranberry	372	Low	53
Grape	253	No Reaction	54
Grapefruit	304	Very Low	55
Lemon	217	No Reaction	56
Orange	233	No Reaction	57
Papaya	215	No Reaction	58
Peach	269	Very Low	59
Pear	147	No Reaction	60
Pineapple	271	Very Low	61
Plum	148	No Reaction	62
Raspberry	201	No Reaction	63
Strawberry	197	No Reaction	64
NUTS/GRAINS			
Almond	797	Moderate	65
Amaranth Flour	298	Very Low	66
Barley	362	Very Low	67
Bean (Kidney)	1685	Very High	68
Bean (Lima)	917	High	69
Bean (Pinto)	1303	High	70
Bean (Soy)	360	Very Low	71
Bean (String)	1437	High	72
Buckwheat	213	No Reaction	73
Coconut	317	Very Low	74
Corn	281	Very Low	75
Filbert	308	Very Low	76
Green Pea	300	Very Low	77
Lentil	212	No Reaction	78
Millet	198	No Reaction	79
Oat	262	No Reaction	80
Peanut	316	Very Low	81
Pecan	263	No Reaction	82
Rice	164	No Reaction	83
Rye	483	Low	84
Sesame	1560	Very High	85
Spelt	267	No Reaction	86
Sunflower	599	Moderate	87
Walnut	1142	High	88
Wheat (Gluten)	274	Very Low	89
Whole Wheat	254	No Reaction	90
MISCELLANY			
Cocoa Bean	1636	Very High	91
Coffee Bean	544	Moderate	92
Honey	616	Moderate	93
Sugar Cane	426	Low	94
Yeast (Baker)	1604	Very High	95
Yeast (Brewer)	1496	High	96

Scale across top: 500 600 700 800 900 1000 1100 1200 1300 1400 1500

High (Very High, Extremely High) IgG reactivity is highlighted with a gray background.

The ELISA analysis is a semi-quantitative assessment for specific IgG antibody levels. This test has not been evaluated by the FDA.

rather a chronic inflammatory reaction. Think of food sensitivity as a conflict of interest: Your epithelial cells are shopping for nutrients at the perimeter of your intestine while your immune system is simultaneously fighting a war in the same place.

This conflict causes the body to miss out on the good nutrition passing through because food is not being absorbed properly. It's like when your inbox is full of spam: too much spam makes it a lot easier to miss the important messages. Eating something that triggers an immune response compromises your body's ability to properly absorb other nutrients. When you stop eating the food that causes this immune response, your gut not only reduces its immune response but is better able to utilize the rest of the essential nutrients in your food.

In my work as a medical adviser to youth sports and to collegiate, Olympic, and professional athletes, both men and women, I've seen great examples of food sensitivity causing nutrients to not be utilized properly. Many athletes are protein-deficient, even though they consume lots of protein, and suffer from mood, energy, and intestinal issues. I've seen numerous athletes with these problems who regularly drink whey-based protein shakes but are still protein deficient. Blood tests often show that they are sensitive to whey/casein. When they switch to pea protein or other non-whey protein smoothies, such as my Organic Super Protein (**www.menoclinic.com/smoothies**) their athletic performance improves, as does their protein absorption, and their issues disappear. These athletes were consuming plenty of protein, but the inflammatory response and resultant state of their intestines made their body unable to utilize the protein properly. The lesson for you is clear: What are you eating that is keeping you from using the nutrients in other foods you eat?

Another problematic response to food messaging happens when fat storage SNPs are turned on (as they are in obese individuals): food is immediately turned into fat. This explains why exercise alone will not cure obesity—if you're obese, your epigenetic markers are telling your metabolic system to convert food to fat, leaving you with little energy to burn yet many thousands of calories packed away in the form of fat. From a nutritional perspective, many obese people are essentially starving within a cocoon of stored calories.

It is through the gut that most people do themselves the most damage, but it is also the place where the solution is most often found. Fully one-third of your genes respond to what you eat. With the wrong information, your genes initiate a response that can cause chronic disease—and may even leave SNPs for chronic disease turned on in the genetic code you pass on to your children. With the right information, your cells manufacture enzymes that improve your cholesterol balance, repair damage to your arterial walls, improve nervous system function, turn off inflammatory SNPs, and change who you are, on a cellular level, for the better.

For the last fifty years, medicine has been dividing the body into smaller and smaller pieces and designing treatments accordingly. All indications suggest that we're going to spend the next fifty years putting the body back together and learning how all its systems function as one. We still don't know everything, but we do know now that what's good for your gut is good for your epigenetic messaging, which is good for your heart, your brain, and every cell in your body—and it all starts with what you eat every day.

Making Music

By now, what you've learned about the complexities of heart health must make the prevention of heart disease seem like a Herculean task. But breaking down heart health into its different factors is arming you with information about your unique self. Don't be intimidated by the magnitude of information—it just helps you get to know yourself a little better. I'm about to give you simple self-care tools, available to virtually everyone, that will dramatically improve your heart health and overall vitality, and this information will help you to best use these tools.

A perfect example of the individualized treatment plan used in functional medicine is my client Gina, who visits a famous clinic for

Protecting the Blood-Brain Barrier

The premise of the Heart Solution for Women is simple: reduce systemic inflammation. Inflammation is the difference between a cell that damages your heart and a cell that nurtures it. Not only does chronic inflammation increase the gut's permeability, but—brace yourself for this one—*the blood-brain barrier also becomes more permeable under the stress of chronic inflammation*. Leaky gut is leaky heart is leaky brain—it's gut inflammation that lights the fire on the heart and on the brain.

Toxins enter the brain during periods of systemic inflammation. Other vascular insults can also break down the blood-brain barrier, which, after all, is merely a robust network of tiny capillaries. We now know what we've suspected for years—as your gut succumbs to inflammation, so does your heart and brain, and as your gut heals, so do your heart and brain.

her executive physical every year. When she came to see me at sixty-eight years of age, she was on two diabetes medicines and a statin drug, but still had dangerous levels of blood sugar and lipids, including cholesterol and triglycerides.

Six months later, she was off all of her medicines and her blood tests showed that her baseline health was better than when she was on the medications. After Gina went for her executive physical that year, her doctor called me and asked, "How in the world did you do this?" I told him about the Precision, Personalized Solution, and he replied, "Well, that will never work on a large scale." I responded, "Well, it's working one person at a time, and if we can do it one person at a time, why can't we do it for a hundred at a time?"

Once you commit to improving your health heart, you'll also benefit from the beautiful music of the pleasant side effects: prevention of heart disease also reduces stress and prevents dementia and Alzheimer's, weight gain, diabetes, and depression. The Precision, Personalized Solution to heart health increases energy, happiness, fitness, body image, sexual satisfaction, self-esteem, confidence, social engagement, and overall vitality, from youth through midlife and into old age.

The heart, the brain, the genes, and the gut—for optimal heart health, all four instruments of the functional medicine quartet must be kept tuned and balanced over an entire lifetime. Falling back into the status quo of mainstream Western food and lifestyle will cause the instruments of your body to fall out of tune and heart health will decline. As in a string quartet, if even one instrument is out of tune, the music from all four sounds bad.

Your self-knowledge is your tuning fork for maintaining the body harmony that is essential for you to resist and reverse heart disease. The more you use your self-knowledge the more your heart heals, and you'll feel it heal, giving you the confidence that nobody in the world is more of an expert about your individual health than you yourself.

Chapter 5

Healing Your Hormones

Your heart health relies on a symphony of information written by the hormonal messaging of the endocrine system. When this symphony is in harmony, you feel great because your hormones are balanced, your immune system is strong, your nutrition is well utilized, it is difficult for disease to take hold, inflammation is low, and you're burning energy efficiently. Your mood is stable and positive, your heart is happy, and vitality is yours to enjoy in every aspect of life. When the symphony is out of balance, however, you're more susceptible to disease, inflammation is high, you store calories more easily than you burn them, your mood is variable or low, your gut is not absorbing nutrition properly, and both your quality of life and heart health suffer. This chapter will give you an "ear" for listening to your hormonal messaging in a more educated way so that you can more effectively heal your particular imbalances with the tools presented in Part III.

I'm still awestruck by the number of times patients have presented with a wide array of issues—including brain fog, depression, high blood pressure, weight problems, and even the beginnings of heart disease and dementia—but then those symptoms improved dramatically when we uncovered the hormonal culprit causing the problems and targeted it with precision, personalized lifestyle medicine. Even more amazingly, not only is their primary complaint resolved, but many other elements of their health improve. That sore knee becomes pain free. Nights are filled with beautiful dreams rather than restless eternities. Brain fog dissipates and gives way to a clear mind. Body weight decreases. Energy improves. Lipid and cholesterol balance improves. Blood pressure decreases. Life. Gets. Better.

To understand how your hormonal symphony functions, let's examine how each of the players in the endocrine system relates to your body's vascular health, inflammation, and ways of exchanging information—your body's hormonal music. It's a complicated relationship, but it boils down to a cycle of information that provides insight into your particular problems and will help you build your own Precision, Personalized Solution.

The Pituitary

The conductor of your body's symphony is the pituitary, a pea-size gland at the base of the brain. Like any good conductor, the pituitary not only commands attention but also listens and adjusts its messaging based on input from the rest of the symphony. The pituitary has been called "the master gland" because, in our early studies of glandular function, it appeared that the hormones produced there controlled the functions of other hormones that regulate metabolism, sexual function, tissues, reproduction, sleep, growth, development, immune response, and more. As with so many stories in medicine, this turned out to be only half of the truth.

The other half was revealed when we learned about the hormonal pathways that drive the pituitary to produce its hormones. The pituitary receives messages in the form of neural and hormonal inputs from other parts of the body, including glands, cells, and the brain. It turns out that the pituitary is not so much a "master gland" as a hormonal switchboard: it receives hormonal information from the farthest reaches of your body, sorts it, then sends it back along the same pathway. This information pathway begins in your gut with the food you eat and the stress, emotions, and external pressures processed by the vast neurological network in your intestines. Carried through your body in ways that are still not entirely understood, these messages not only influence your organs and functions but also, like gossipy teenagers at the mall, have pronounced effects on the secretions and actions of other hormones.

In spite of its great influence on the body's diverse systems, the pituitary's own blood supply is incredibly fragile compared to that of a robust organ like the heart. A history of head injuries, particularly concussions, can have a dramatic impact on the functioning of the pituitary, and therefore all of the downstream hormones in the endocrine symphony. This is one reason why repeated concussions can cause a wide range of issues in systems related to the pituitary, and also why hormone replacement therapies for pituitary gland function seem to improve function in individuals who have suffered a traumatic brain injury. You don't have to be fully knocked unconscious after a head injury to suffer a concussion; new research shows that damage from even minor trauma to the head can cause long-term issues.

Many women will tell you, "I was never the same after the birth of my child." One of these changes that relates most to heart health is the effect of childbirth on the pituitary. Because your blood volume doubles during pregnancy and then half of it is lost in seconds during birth, the pituitary, with its fragile blood supply, can be "starved" for blood and nourishment. The pituitary of a woman with a healthy heart can recover, but a compromised heart doesn't support recovery as well as a strong one. Sheehan's syndrome—the pituitary equivalent of a heart attack—is a serious condition in which lack of blood flow to the pituitary following childbirth causes total pituitary failure. When your pituitary isn't functioning well, your entire symphony suffers.

Far too often in medicine we think of function as "all or nothing," but one of the things I hope to convey in this book is the importance of also paying attention to "relative dysfunction." Relative dysfunction is when your lab tests are "normal" but you certainly don't feel normal. Slightly decreased efficiency in the pituitary is a good example: very small amounts of hormones can have incredible downstream effects. The amount of hormone in your blood is a speck of sand according to test results, but the effect on your mood and energy can feel like a boulder.

The Thyroid

The thyroid could be called your energy gland. Some of the thyroid hormones' most important functions are to help convert food into energy, regulate body heat, and boost metabolism in your muscles' mitochondria, the power plants in your cells.

Hypothyroidism, a health problem caused by low levels of thyroid hormone, is a common cause of dangerous levels of cholesterol and other lipids. This happens when levels of thyroid hormones, which regulate the liver's cholesterol production, fall and the liver produces excess cholesterol. At the same time, your metabolism slows and your internal temperature drops—a perfect storm for fat storage and hormonal imbalance. The temperature change is slight, but the consequences are significant. Proteins must be folded into a perfect shape for optimal function, and to fold perfectly they need to form at that optimal temperature of 98.6 degrees Fahrenheit. When proteins are formed into their most efficient structure at the right temperature, they open up the metabolic pathway—the delivery mechanism for energy, nutrients, and hormones, including the thyroid hormones that affect every tissue in your body. Cholesterol uses proteins in order to travel through your bloodstream to the tissues where it is needed. When the proteins take on a different shape because they were formed at a lower temperature, the cholesterol trying to bond with the misshapen proteins also takes on different, and more detrimental, characteristics.

Have you ever heard that little voice inside your head whisper, "Are my hormones making it difficult for me to lose weight?"

If so, the little voice may be right, and probably because of compromised thyroid function. In the named dysfunction associated with this phenomenon, Wilson's temperature syndrome, the individual has decreased thyroid function, dangerously high cholesterol levels, and low body temperature. Obesity and easy weight gain are closely associated with Wilson's temperature syndrome, and the root of the problem is the thyroid. With thyroid deficiency, your entire metabolic system suffers and your "bad" cholesterol increases.

This is where the oversimplified concept of "bad" and "good" cholesterol comes from—when cholesterol is optimized for use by your tissues, it's a good thing, but when it's not delivered, or delivered by improperly formed proteins, or left to accumulate in chronically inflamed areas of your vascular system, cholesterol takes on "bad" characteristics. This is what we're talking about in functional medicine circles when we say, "You are your cholesterol." We all have cholesterol, lots of it, and we can make more if we need it, but what matters is the kind of cholesterol we have. Thyroid function is one of the primary factors in determining whether your cholesterol is the "good" kind— the big and fluffy particles that protect your heart—or the small and sticky "bad" kind that contributes to heart disease.

Thyroid function also partly explains why the status quo approach to cholesterol management (recommending less dietary fat and more drugs) has gotten it so wrong. If your doctor prescribes cholesterol-lowering medication to treat your high cholesterol, your cholesterol will almost certainly decrease, and your doctor will consider your case a success, but your root problem will not change: cholesterol-lowering medications do nothing to restore proper thyroid function. To complicate matters further, as these statin drugs negatively affect the mitochondria energy factories in your muscles, your thyroid function is likely to decrease and your core issues will only worsen.

Identifying thyroid dysfunction isn't really that difficult, but it takes time, information, and awareness of the symptoms for a doctor to diagnose it. The Precision, Personalized Solution includes a self-test for thyroid issues as well as thyroid-specific therapies.

The Adrenal

The adrenal is your hero gland, known for producing the stuff that adventure, near misses, and legends are made of—adrenaline. Not as well known are the adrenal hormones that regulate how your body converts fats, proteins, and carbohydrates into energy. If the adrenal gland isn't functioning optimally, you'll have either too much circulating blood sugar or too little. The stress response of the adrenal gland also narrows your blood vessels and increases your blood pressure—not a good thing if you live in a constant state of stress.

The adrenal hormones help regulate your response to environmental stress, including your immune response. One of the most crucial roles of the adrenal gland is to suppress inflammatory response; if your adrenal gland's capacity to suppress inflammation is compromised, your immune system damages your body and your long-term prognosis is grim indeed.

Adrenal health is controversial, thanks to misunderstandings about an officially unrecognized condition, adrenal fatigue, and two recognized conditions, adrenal insufficiency and adrenal crisis. Adrenal insufficiency and crisis are often related to Addison's disease, a condition in which the adrenal glands are damaged and do not produce enough cortisol. As a result, the individual suffers long-lasting fatigue, muscle weakness, loss of appetite, pain in the abdomen, and unwanted weight loss. Adrenal insufficiency and crisis can be diagnosed through blood and saliva tests. There is no conclusive test for adrenal fatigue, but in my observation it is a very real issue.

I like to think of adrenal fatigue as something more like adrenal "dysregulation." What happens is that the adrenal gland gets whipped around and thrown out of its rhythm every time your blood sugar has a major shift, whether high or low. Most hormones have a daily rhythm, female hormones have a monthly rhythm as well, and it's likely that many hormones have seasonal and lifetime rhythms that we don't even understand yet. When the adrenal is functioning with optimum rhythm, it produces cortisol strategically, which increases energy levels to get you out of bed, peaks during midday for optimal energy during the late afternoon and early evening, and finally decreases in the evening to allow deep restorative sleep.

If your sleep is poor, you probably have some form of adrenal dysregulation. During the thirty-six-hour shifts I worked during my internal medicine residency, I was awake the whole time, taking care of very sick people every three days for nearly four years. Do you think my adrenals were "dysregulated"? Absolutely. Perhaps this is why medical students experience up to 50 percent depression rates and more than a 40 percent divorce rate.

I am sure I was mildly depressed during my residency. I put on 15 pounds of extra fat eating pizza during lunch and didn't dream at all during sleep. I had elevated blood pressure and my doctor recommended medication to lower it. Today, at age fifty-five, I am the fittest I have ever been, I sleep great, and I'm happy and healthy. This is one of the benefits I want to share with you about the Heart Solution for Women: you may sign up for optimal heart health and heart attack prevention, but you will leave with more energy, less pain, no brain fog, improved sleep, and a sense of vitality every day!

Every major stress in your life affects your adrenal health. The key to healing is balancing this stress to allow the adrenals to "re-regulate." I will show you how to assess and address adrenal imbalance in Chapter 6, but for now, the simplest recipe for adrenal health is this: fermented foods combined with low sugar consumption makes for happy adrenals. Fermented foods are a prebiotic that feeds the probiotic helpers in your gut, which in turn reduce the bad bacteria, giving your immune response a break. A low-sugar and low-carbohydrate diet will also encourage healthy gut bacteria by preventing the whipping around of the adrenals with high and low blood sugar, and reducing the inflammatory insulin response—effectively lowering the adrenal gland's overall inflammation suppression workload.

The Gonadal

As we've talked about, the statistical variability in heart disease risk between men and women is partly due to the protective quality of women's sex hormones before menopause. Unfortunately, as you well know by now, women's lower early risk of heart disease has resulted in you, my dear reader, getting shortchanged by the medical community, which has essentially said, "Women have less chance of heart disease, so we don't need to worry about them."

Before menopause, estrogen does offer some protection against heart disease, but the protective effect disappears after menopause. Although the exact reason for this protection isn't well understood, researchers point to the fact that estrogen increases HDL (good) cholesterol levels.

The other forgotten fact about women's heart risk is that any hormone—particularly synthetic hormones from birth control, hormone therapy, fertility drugs, and even some nutritional supplements—can increase their blood clot risk for stroke and heart attack prior to menopause. There are specific genetic risk factors that make some women particularly susceptible to this risk, and we always check those in my clinic before prescribing any type of hormones. If a woman has a very high genetic risk for hormone imbalance, then we do everything possible to avoid synthetic hormones of any kind, and if we do use hormones, we are extra vigilant about testing and monitoring.

There are other theories as to why estrogen helps protect against heart disease. Estrogen is involved in the regulation of genes that have cardioprotective (heart protection) qualities, is beneficial to mitochondrial (muscle energy) function, bolsters the function of the essential endothelial layer lining the arteries, and is even associated with reduced blood pressure. In other words, when it comes to protecting the heart, the hormone estrogen verges on the magical.

Regardless of the reason, estrogen's near-magical shield unfortunately has reinforced heart medicine's historical bias against women, relative lack of knowledge about heart disease in women, and naive undertreatment of it. As I mentioned earlier, if a husband and wife go to the emergency room after dinner, both complaining of chest pains, it would not be unusual for the doctor to check him for a heart attack—and give her heartburn medication (ignoring her heart entirely). New research suggests, however, that in the presence of ovarian deficiency (menopause or premature menopause), women's risk from heart health threats like obesity, insulin overproduction, and high cholesterol and blood pressure is equal to men's. We're all terrified of breast cancer, but in fact more women die from cardiovascular disease in the United States than from any other cause. I have no hesitation in saying that the biggest ball the medical community has ever dropped—in part because of the misleading data on the protective qualities of estrogen—is women's heart health.

Testosterone plays a role also, helping to manage abdominal fat through better metabolism of lipids, and starchy carbohydrates. In short, sex hormones interact with the body in ways far more complex than simply driving sex and childbirth. For decades we've known that defective genetic mutations in sex hormones reduce arterial function, specifically in that key endothelial layer where inflammation, nutrient exchange, and plaque formation occur. In the brain, sex hormones act like steroids, influencing mood, learning, memory, and our reaction to rewards. And get this—there are even sex hormone receptors in the heart muscle.

The crucial message here is that proper levels of sex hormones optimize your body in a way that supports robust heart health. As a man, I need a bit of female estrogen—but not too much. As a woman, you need a small amount of testosterone, but again, not too much. And just as too much testosterone could be problematic for me, you also don't want too much estrogen. The key for women is to have a balance between estrogen and its partner, progesterone. Estrogen dominance is when estrogen levels get too high in relation to progesterone; sabotaging all other hormonal systems, it is often missed by doctors.

The delicate nature of hormone balance is why eating meat or dairy products produced from animals treated with hormones is detrimental to your heart. These xenoestrogens mimic estrogens and are found throughout the environment. Bisphenol A, for instance, is in many plastics and binds to cells in a way that increases heart disease (and cancer) risk. Defenders of xenoestrogen use argue that there are only small amounts of xenoestrogens in hormone-treated food products, but even a small amount of hormonal influence, especially when ingested throughout a lifetime, can cause problems. Also, products marketed as herbal hormone supplements may in fact have the opposite effect from what's advertised. It's important not to undertake any kind of hormone supplement therapy without consulting a trusted doctor who has expertise in hormonal treatments and tests for hormone levels before prescribing hormone supplements. And perhaps most importantly, listen to your intuition: if you're like every other woman I see in my clinic, there's a good chance you already know what you need.

The Second Brain

As mentioned earlier, the gut has been called the "second brain" because of its incredible control over bodily function through the vast network of neurons lining and surrounding the intestines. Much of the breakthrough medicine in recent years (and of the near future, I'd predict) has been based on manipulating the neurological functioning of the intestines.

Peptides, hormones that originate in the gut, are some of the more mysterious elements of the body's endocrine system. There is some evidence that peptides directly influence brain function in dramatic ways, but our current understanding of the brain–gut hormone relationship is rudimentary at best. We do know that peptides act in two distinctly different roles: they carry messages, like true hormones, through the bloodstream, and they also hang out on the surface of receiving cells to stimulate their function.

Peptides play a role in your ability to control how much you eat by sending messages to your brain that you are either hungry or satiated. They signal growth hormone production and have positive effects on cardiovascular output. Peptides also regulate and respond to fluctuations in stomach acid—too much of which causes ulcers, and too little of which lets nutrients slip through undigested. They also control the pace of digestion by interacting with the muscles that push chyme (partially digested food) through your intestines.

Weight gain and fat utilization are directly related to peptides. Experiments immunizing rats against production of certain peptides have resulted in decreased weight gain and fat deposition. The influence of peptides on weight gain is so dramatic that researchers have suggested that manipulation of peptides could result in a vaccine against obesity.

Peptide-based therapies are also revealing exciting potential for other disease prevention, including that of cancer and arthritis as well as heart disease. Researchers in multiple studies have voiced the opinion that peptide therapy shows great promise, but caution that many studies are in the early stage and more data are needed before specific treatments can be used for human health. Antioxidant vitamins—beneficial due in part to their positive effect on peptides—were traditionally considered safe even in high doses, but recent research has shown that taking high-dose antioxidants can increase disease risk or cause an allergic response in some people. (Once again, we don't all respond the same!)

One day we may have a miracle pharmaceutical that balances hormones, but for now, not wanting to wait around, we can turn to diet, lifestyle, nutritional supplements, and, if necessary, pharmaceuticals to optimize the biochemistry of our hormonal information network. While the science is still evolving, there is no question as to the enormous influence of hormones on heart health, and we can be certain that anything that throws hormones out of balance will increase the risk of heart disease.

When I consider the symphony of true health and look at the external factors that may be contributing to hormonal imbalance and elevated heart disease risk, I always consider four sources of damage: food, toxins, bugs, and trauma. We've already talked about how food influences biochemistry and heart disease risk, so let's look at toxins, bugs, and trauma.

Toxins

Everyone loves to talk about toxins, but few define what kind of toxin they're talking about. Essentially, a toxin is a poison. There are toxins in the environment as well as naturally occurring toxins produced in our bodies that are toxic only if they move to where they're not supposed to be. Environmental toxins are all around us, and their influence on heart disease is dramatic, but science has yet to explain exactly why. In trying to prevent and reverse heart disease, however, we don't need to know why—just knowing that toxins can cause heart disease is enough. For now, let's focus on environmental toxins.

Alcohol

Alcohol may be the most famous toxin in human history. My opinion is that we're still waiting for the final verdict on whether low levels of alcohol are beneficial. I don't like to use the term "moderate" when talking about alcohol consumption. In practice, it's too easy to let "moderate" slip into "moderately drunk." I think of alcohol consumption relative to the individual: just because some study shows that a couple of glasses of wine are beneficial for an Italian living on the Mediterranean doesn't mean that a couple of glasses of wine each night will be beneficial for me, an Italian living in Wyoming. I would caution that the health problems of even moderate wine consumption likely outweigh the benefits.

The 2015–2020 US Dietary Guidelines for Americans recommends maximum consumption of one drink per day for women and two for men (emerging data indicates that these recommendations are probably too high). Have one drink as per day and *you might* receive some heart health benefit. Suck down that second one and you've negated any benefit from the first one as well as increased your risk of heart disease.

One of the theories about red wine is that its beneficial qualities stem from resveratrol, a plant compound with anti-inflammatory and antioxidant qualities, but the data haven't really supported this theory. Resveratrol occurs in such low amounts in red wine that it is unlikely to have therapeutic benefit and one study found that blood resveratrol levels have nothing to do with disease development anyway. To put the potential resveratrol benefit from red wine in perspective, a therapeutic dose of resveratrol is about 20 milligrams, a dose that would require drinking 41 glasses of wine to achieve—a deadly way to get your resveratrol. Studies have shown that people who drink wine have higher levels of HDL (good) cholesterol than people who don't drink wine (but maybe that's because wine drinkers eat more healthy fats). The naturally occurring anti-inflammatories and antioxidants in wine may provide benefit, but to confuse the issue further, another study showed that the health benefit of one drink per day is the same for all types of alcohol, not just for wine. (But the study included zero women, so like many studies on heart disease, it may mean absolutely nothing to you.)

Liquor is hardest on your liver, and beer and mixed drinks have the highest carbohydrate/sugar content, so wine may be the healthiest in this regard. In my office, I have a picture of a wineglass full of sugar with a little yeast sprinkled on it. I tell all my patients trying to lose weight or avoid alcohol to go home, fill a wineglass with sugar, and remember each time they drink a glass of wine that they're consuming a glass of sugar. It's not that wine has a sugar content equivalent to a full glass of sugar, but the metabolic and toxic effect of consuming the sugars, alcohol, and empty carbohydrates in a glass of wine is comparable to consuming a glass of sugar.

Another reason to take studies demonstrating the health benefits of alcohol with a grain of salt is the difficulty of statistically separating alcohol consumption from other lifestyle factors. It could be that red wine has been shown to be more beneficial simply because those who drink red wine may also exercise more, buy healthier foods, and have more social support because they're enjoying a meal with friends as they drink wine. The results may have nothing to do with the wine at all! Also, numerous studies demonstrating the health benefits of alcohol were funded by the alcohol industry. This doesn't mean the science is wrong, but it does mean the fox is sleeping awfully close to the henhouse. Just because the people chosen for a study benefited from one drink per day doesn't mean you will.

Alcohol damages your liver, is toxic to the wiring of your heart, and can cause a deadly rhythm abnormality called atrial fibrillation. It also reduces the number of oxygen-carrying red blood cells and substantially increases your risk of certain types of cancers. Heavy drinking is particularly damaging because it causes blood to clot, which increases the chance of heart attack and stroke, as well as shrinkage in certain areas of the brain. Studies have shown that middle-aged people who drink heavily are three times more likely to develop dementia and Alzheimer's. One study demonstrated that alcohol abuse increases the risk of heart problems, including heart attack, heart rhythm abnormalities, and congestive heart failure, as much as any other risk factor for heart disease, including high blood pressure, smoking, diabetes, and obesity.

Here's the bottom line for your own Precision, Personalized Solution: the data aren't conclusive enough for me to say with confidence that one drink per day is good for you; what I can say, however, is that if you don't drink, don't start drinking with the idea that it will protect your heart!

Smoking

Everyone knows they should exercise, lose weight, and stop smoking. But it wasn't always this way. My favorite slide during my presentation for medical conferences is a 1940s magazine ad for cigarettes showing a doctor in his white coat smoking at his desk with the caption: "More doctors choose Camel than any other cigarette." When I was five years old, I remember, the pediatrician for my kindergarten wellness visit examined me with a cigarette dangling out of his mouth, reeking of smoke, and with an ashtray full of cigarette butts on his desk! To this day cigarette smoke makes me ill.

Remember how people used to smoke on airplanes? As if the air quality on planes isn't bad enough! It is mind-boggling to imagine this happening now, but what if we're making equally counterproductive assumptions today about the healthiness of other behavior? What if this is where we are now with some of our medications—as ignorant about the dangers of some of the drugs and food products we're using as doctors were in the '60s about smoking?

A million words have been written about the dangers of smoking, and I don't think I can put it any more clearly. But in my clinic, if you are an active smoker, you can't come back unless you at least sign a contract with me with a timeline and plan to quit smoking. Maybe this seems harsh, but if you're smoking I can't help you. There is no intervention or therapy anyone can do for you that will outweigh the damaging effects and oxidized stress caused by smoking. Studies show that, for rats, nicotine is more addictive than heroin! Smokers who undergo plastic surgery do not heal as well as nonsmokers. Most of my plastic surgeon friends will not take a client who smokes—they know the skin doesn't heal as well, the outcome will not be optimal, and the client's smoking will counteract the amazing work they do.

If you make the commitment to quit, I can tell you that the challenge to quit smoking is dramatically easier when accompanied by other lifestyle and diet changes that support improved health. I tell my patients that it takes only seventy-two hours to break the addiction and twenty-one days to change the habit. To help people quit, we give them a road map that shows them how to identify and break the links in their chain of smoking. It works.

Stop smoking now. You won't regret it. And once you have quit for ten years, you'll have the same low cancer risk that I do having never smoked—except the passive smoke I got from my pediatrician!

Heavy Metals

The world would be a much healthier place if heavy metal stayed on the stage as a musical genre rather than infiltrating our water supply, food sources, and even nutritional supplements. Himalayan sea salt is a good source of the mineral because it was formed millions of years ago when those mountains were covered by oceans and long before we poisoned our world with heavy metals. This is also why taking coral calcium as a support for your bone health should be avoided—it is harvested from coral reefs, which are loaded with heavy metals, just like most of the fish in our oceans.

The mechanism of damage to our bodies caused by heavy metals—lead, arsenic, cadmium, and mercury—is not entirely understood, but the cutting-edge best guess is that it's related to how heavy metals alter genetic expression, acting essentially like a computer virus in our genetic microprocessors. Heavy metals may also function like "gas on the fire" of cellular inflammation in your arteries, making any plaque much more likely to rupture and kill you.

Numerous studies have connected elevated heavy metal levels with increased heart disease risk, and lead and arsenic have been linked to high blood pressure (and cancer) for decades, but unfortunately these findings are overshadowed by the hyperbole surrounding heavy metals and their impact on human health. Anyone who's paid attention to health news over the last thirty years will remember the frenzy of throwing out aluminum cookware for fear of the metal causing Alzheimer's. As it turns out, studies have not shown any increased dementia risk from using aluminum cookware, probably because the form of aluminum in cookware is not as bioavailable (absorbable by your cells) as other forms of the metal. But before you cook tonight's dinner in that aluminum pan, consider how much easier it is to burn food in a thin aluminum pan than it is in a heavy cast-iron or stainless steel pan—and that charred food does have proven carcinogenic properties. There are good reasons to avoid using thin aluminum pans, but the danger of ingesting the aluminum isn't one of them.

The studies that caused the aluminum cookware hysteria were initially thought to be a smoking gun connecting aluminum to Alzheimer's because pathology reports on the brains of those who had died from Alzheimer's showed aluminum deposition. A pathology review shows, however, that Alzheimer's brains show elevations of all heavy metals, and other heavy metals are commonly found in chemical forms that are far more bioavailable than aluminum. Lead, by comparison, is readily absorbed and is still exceedingly common in our human environment. The dangers of heavy metals are a major reason for Proposition 65, the California legislation requiring that many of the products sold in the state carry warning labels about their associated health risks.

The average American woman is exposed to 168 different chemicals before leaving the house in the morning. Sure, a lot of them have been designated as safe; others, however, are considered safe in America but not in other countries, still others have not been tested for human safety, and some are just plain toxic. A recent study revealed that women with darker skin are at higher risk for toxicity from cosmetics than women with lighter skin. The pigments used in makeup for darker skin, the cultural pressures on women with darker skin, and the relative scarcity of less toxic options have combined to elevate the risk. Skin Deep, a database on personal care products, reports that blood from a group of teenagers was found to contain sixteen hormone-altering chemicals that came from cosmetics and other products applied to the skin.

The regulated limits on heavy metals in cosmetics vary dramatically between countries. In Germany, the limit for lead is two parts per million (2PPM). In Canada, the limit is 10 PPM. In the United States, the FDA has no authority to enforce heavy metal limits in cosmetics but has recommended a limit on par with Canada's 10 PPM.

(Let's see, what's the score now? Women get short changed by heart research, shamed into dieting even when they have healthy body weight, have their heart attacks confused with heartburn and treated counterproductively, and are sold toxins in beauty products. I'm so sorry. I hope I'm helping to right some of these wrongs by pouring everything I know about women's heart health into the pages of this book. Back to the toxins.)

In 2012, the news of arsenic in rice delivered a crushing blow to fans of Asian cuisine and health food enthusiasts who saw rice as a healthier alternative to pasta and other, more processed carbohydrates. If the world's rice supply is contaminated with arsenic from pesticides and poultry fertilizer, what can we eat? It's a serious question that doesn't bode well for the future of the world's food supply. Heavy metals have also been found in certified organic foods, vitamins, dietary supplements, and herbs.

The sad truth is that, no matter where we go or what we eat, we can't avoid ingesting heavy metals. But we can minimize our exposure to these toxins and the damage they cause.

If you eat a variety of all types of food, you minimize your chance of eating a lot of any one kind or brand that has exceptionally high heavy metal content. Avoid using products and taking supplements you don't need. Everything from prescription and over-the-counter drugs, baby formula, hair products, and skin cream to ceramics, and refined chocolate can contain high levels of heavy metals.

Ten years ago, I was told that everyone with metal fillings in their cavities should have their fillings removed due to the risk of heavy metal poisoning from mercury. I didn't really believe it until I visited Sam Queen, one of the gurus in mercury toxicity, at the Institute for Health Realities. His expertise comes from personal experience, not just education and theory. He was poisoned by mercury in a freak lab accident. The exposure was so intense that his lab partner died soon after. Sam cured himself with organic foods, clean distilled water, and natural chelation.

I talked to patients of his who had been wheelchair-bound with what was diagnosed as multiple sclerosis. After undergoing chelation therapy to remove heavy metals from their brains and nervous systems, they were able to go running on the beach. During my cardiology rotation while training at the VA hospital in Phoenix, I saw patients whose heart disease had made them barely able to walk, but who became joggers after chelation therapy—and no other heart interventions—for calcium deposits in their hearts.

The government has finally taken notice. The National Institutes of Health's recently completed Trial to Assess Chelation Therapy (TACT), which evaluated chelation's effects on cardiovascular disease, showed a modest benefit. (As a side note, that a government study on chelation therapy actually showed a benefit was shocking to every doctor who read it, as most thought the idea of chelation for heart

How to Avoid Arsenic

Arsenic in rice is an example of the importance of frequently and diligently researching the latest information on the foods you eat. Consider the following to minimize your arsenic exposure due to rice consumption:

- White rice contains less arsenic than brown rice.

- Processed rice food products contain more arsenic than plain rice.

- Rinsing the rice thoroughly and cooking the rice in extra water (6 cups of water for every 1 cup of rice) has been shown to remove 35 to 45 percent of the arsenic from the rice.

- Rice cakes have exceptionally high arsenic content.

- Rice from California, Pakistan, and India has the least arsenic.

- Rice from US states other than California—especially Arkansas, Louisiana, and Texas—has the most arsenic.

disease was a scam. Well, it does work—*but not for everybody!* This is the problem with the "one size fits all" medicine we're taught in medical school. Perhaps those who don't benefit have poor gut health and can't excrete the heavy metals after chelation, or perhaps their underfunctioning liver is overwhelmed and unable to deal with further strain. Recognizing these possibilities is the "secret sauce" of functional medicine—everyone is unique, and an individual's therapy should be adjusted to their physiology for optimal outcomes.)

How do we make sense of the recommendation to remove our fillings? Well, if we were all highly and equally sensitive to heavy metal toxicity, everyone with mercury/silver amalgam fillings would be wheelchair-bound with MS, but we're not. It's not that heavy metals don't cause MS—they likely do—but that individual sensitivity to these substances varies and we don't know what an individual's tolerance for heavy metals will be. Some people are the metaphorical canary in the coal mine, while others can handle incredible levels of heavy metal toxicity without obvious damage. At the VA hospital, I saw men who could barely walk down the hall. Six months later, after thirty rounds of chelation therapy from an alternative medicine doctor, they could walk three miles. I also saw men who could barely walk down the hall, who got thirty rounds of chelation, and afterwards could still barely walk down the hall. We don't all respond the same to toxins and we don't all respond the same to therapy.

I hate to say it, but the world's toxicity is increasing to the point where doctors will soon be suggesting that everyone go through an annual or even biannual detox, like your fall and spring house cleanings or your dental checkups. Many people have done a juice fast or "natural cleanse" that tasted lousy and made them feel horrible. In our clinic, we use the Meno Cleanse, which I do quarterly. All of my staff use it as well, because they love it and feel good afterwards, and all of us already eat clean and watch toxins like hawks. The Meno Cleanse (www.menoclinic.com/cleanse) is a packaged and premixed meal plan: You drink a tasty, easy-to-use, and fruity protein smoothie for breakfast and lunch that contains all of the nutrients to support the liver, the gut, and the detox process. Then you have a clean dinner with your family, which we show you how to easily shop for and prepare in a healthy way. See—a cleanse doesn't have to be hard or taste horrible or alienate you from the family meal!

In our toxin-laden world, everyone, whatever their baseline health or lifestyle, needs to detox. A detox program needs to be intensive and effective but doesn't have to be unpleasant—you don't have to have pain to get the gain. Find a healthy, safe, gentle-yet-effective detox, especially the first time, and do it under the supervision of a physician, not a fringe specialist.

Bugs

For eons, we weren't afraid of the tiniest bugs because we didn't know they existed. Then, three hundred years ago, Antonie van Leeuwenhoek invented the microscope and for the next two hundred years we were afraid of bugs because we knew they were killing us and we couldn't do anything about it. A hundred years ago, Alexander Fleming discovered penicillin, and once again we weren't afraid of bugs because we had antibiotics to chase them away. Now we should be scared of bugs again.

Here's why. Traditional risk factors for atherosclerosis (hardening of the arteries) include hypertension (high blood pressure), hyperlipidemia (high cholesterol and high triglycerides), gender (men have higher risk across all age groups), diabetes, tobacco use, and family history. We've known for some time, however, that these factors account for only half of the clinical cases of atherosclerosis. So what causes the other half?

As we're now learning, things that affect one part of your body don't affect it in isolation. Polymerase chain reaction (PCR) technology—the same technology used to track criminals by examining the DNA left at a crime scene (think *CSI*, the TV show)—has shed a disturbing light on that other 50 percent. DNA from one type of the bacteria chlamydia (not the same as the lung infection or the STD) has been found by PCR in atherosclerosis and thrombotic plaques in the heart. Another PCR study on vascular walls found *Chlamydia pneumoniae* DNA in 26 percent of the atherosclerotic specimens but no *C. pneumoniae* DNA in the healthy vascular wall specimens. In Turkey, where traditional risk factors for heart disease are exceedingly low, there is a high prevalence of heart disease as well as a high rate of infection. We don't know exactly how it works, but it is blindingly clear that chronic infection can cause heart disease.

A really good reason to see a doctor as soon as you suspect an infection is that prompt and aggressive treatment of bacterial infections appears to reduce the risk to your heart. Not all infections that affect vascular health are media darlings like *C. pneumoniae.* Even the humble bacterial infections of the mouth have been linked to heart disease. People with periodontal disease are twice as likely to have heart disease as those with healthy gums. I know what you're thinking: "Aha! Plaque on the teeth causes plaques in the heart!" It's not that simple. There is a link between dental health and vascular health, but it has nothing to do with the plaque on your teeth. Rather, it's that bacterial infection can make its way from the mouth into arterial plaques by way of the bloodstream. We can't say with absolute certainty whether the increase in heart disease is caused by the periodontal bacteria, by the body's inflammatory response to the bacteria, or by a greater susceptibility to periodontal disease in the presence of hardening of the arteries.

From my lifetime of studying health through the diverse lenses of different specialties, observing the body's immune reaction and the proliferation of cellular inflammation, I'd put my money on the inflammatory and information response to bacterial disease as a primary driver of increased heart disease risk. And it seems that other doctors would too: from the Mayo Clinic to the American Diabetes Association, respected medical institutions are recommending that oral hygiene be included in a comprehensive plan for heart health (and brain health).

Then there are the bugs in your gut. For years, functional medicine doctors only whispered about leaky gut and intestinal permeability (to avoid getting yelled at by their attending physicians the way I was), but now everyone is talking about it. There are as many bacterial cells in your gut as there are human cells in your entire body. Half of the DNA inside you is not yours but that of the bugs living in the microbiome of your gut. When your gut becomes permeable due to chronic inflammation, some of these bugs make their way into your bloodstream and into your heart, and their DNA may even penetrate the sacred neurons of your brain. Can these bugs affect your heart health? Without a doubt.

Trauma

When we consider trauma as it relates to heart disease, we're not talking about dramatic injuries like a compound fracture with a broken bone protruding through the skin. We're talking about trauma within your hormonal and vascular systems. Modern medicine can handle acute injuries like a compound fracture, but this less tangible trauma—which is much more subtle, but every bit as dangerous—can be harder to treat.

Coronary artery disease can typically be tracked to an injury of the innermost layer of the coronary artery, deep inside the heart. This injury could have been caused by lack of exercise, extremely high cholesterol, chronic high blood pressure, insulin resistance or diabetes, radiation therapy to the chest, or smoking or secondhand smoke. These injuries can begin as early as childhood.

Women who read heart health books may not be surprised by these possible sources of trauma to the heart, but there's another kind of trauma we don't tend to mention in the conversation about heart disease: the emotional trauma of adverse childhood experiences. Studies have linked these experiences to a variety of adult health conditions, ranging from migraines to depression to heart disease, especially for women.

We use a tool called the ACE (Adverse Childhood Experiences) Score to assess historical physical and emotional trauma. Such trauma doesn't damage the arteries directly, but rather indirectly through its effect on the hormonal stress response and subsequent inflammation. You may tell yourself that past emotional trauma is water under the bridge, but the biochemical changes that happened at that time of severe emotional stress may have had long-lasting effects on your fight-or-flight endocrine system, driving inflammation all over your body that culminates decades later in the form of reduced vitality and increased heart disease risk.

The good news is that while negative childhood experiences increase disease risk later in life, positive experiences in early life build resilience and help protect you from the effects of childhood trauma. There is no official "Positive Childhood Experiences Score" yet; such an assessment tool would almost certainly show that the good things that happen to you early in life reduce your heart disease risk later in life. Having a trusted friend with whom you can share feelings and experiences, unconditional love from a grandparent, or a teacher who believes in you may mitigate the effects of early physical and emotional trauma enough to prevent the adulthood outcome of heart disease.

Trauma is the likely culprit behind the occasional marathon runner who drops dead from a heart attack. Trauma is what ultimately causes both heart attack and stroke. An injury to the artery is most commonly caused by chronic inflammation resulting from a variety of biochemical factors, but it can also be caused by acute physical trauma, such as an injury from a car crash, a sports injury, or even a less dramatic event, like an extreme yoga move, violent vomiting, or a forceful cough. Many of these traumas heal quietly, sometimes incompletely, and you never even realize they happened.

Whatever the cause, the body responds the same with any injury—by sending clotting and repair cells to the injury site. To repair inflammatory injury, your body produces cholesterol and homocysteine to patch it, creating plaques that act like your body's arterial Band-Aids. If the arteries are flexible, healthy, and relatively injury free, this patching method works great. The exterior walls of the artery expand to accommodate the volume of the plaque, and the plaque hardens and creates a new interior wall. The problems occur when the arteries are stiff and cannot expand, and when the plaques are unstable because they're a poor mix of cholesterol types that eventually rupture. Unstable arterial plaques (made up of cholesterol) are like poorly mixed concrete (made up of sand, water, and cement): both were made with the right ingredients, but both are extremely weak because those ingredients weren't mixed in the right proportions.

As you know from Chapter 2, plaque rupture initiates a clotting response from the blood. If the clotting response is not regulated by anticoagulants like omega-3, or if disruptors like lipoprotein-a prevent regulation, the clotting reaction blocks the artery. If the blockage is in arteries that delivered blood to the heart, you have a heart attack. If the blockage is in the arteries that deliver blood to the brain, you have a stroke.

Vascular trauma can also be chronic and develop over many years in the smallest capillaries that feed blood into the brain. Such trauma reduces the oxygen available to the brain and causes prolonged hypoxia. Hypoxia is what can happen to high-altitude mountaineers, but returning to a lower altitude gives them immediate relief.

Some types of vascular trauma can be reversed with lifestyle and dietary changes; more severe cases respond to properly applied supplements and drugs, and in the most extreme cases surgery may be needed. The key lesson here is that vascular trauma is not black-and-white but rather a continuum that begins with easily reversible symptoms (like slightly elevated LDL "bad" cholesterol) and progresses through more-difficult-to-reverse symptoms (like insulin sensitivity) to irreversible disease (like a heart attack).

Power to the Individual

Now you're ready. You've learned about the interconnectedness of your body, the mechanisms at work in it, and the unique involvement of your hormones, and it's time to start healing *you*. Yes, you. The unique you. Maybe you're suffering from a heart disease diagnosis as you read this. Maybe you have been diagnosed with another disease and are worried about your risk. Maybe you're simply worried about developing disease in the future and are concerned about your overall health. Regardless of where you are right now in your functional medicine journey, the program I offer you in Part III can help. The Precision, Personalized Solution is full of ways to tailor your individual risk, intolerances, preferences, and lifestyle to dramatically improve your chance of living a disease-free life.

As an internal medicine doctor in a world where double-blind, placebo-controlled, randomized, multi-centered clinical trials reign supreme, I sometimes wish I could just quote a study that shows the effectiveness of getting your symphony of health into optimal functioning condition. Unfortunately, that's not how individualized health works—and it's not how clinical trials and evidence-based medicine work either. Individualized health care isn't easy for doctors. You don't want to be a unique individual regressed to the mean of a population's bell-shaped curve just to make your doctor's job easy. In clinical trials, one goal is to have a large number of individuals in each group of the trial. This is called the N number, and it's used to give statistical power to the conclusions drawn about the differences between the groups. The larger a study's N (some studies have thousands of people) the more trust you can have in its conclusion—the greater its statistical power.

What functional medicine doctors do is look at those studies for overall guidance but use the N of 1 in the clinic. The idea is to treat you as the individual you are, with your unique genetics, microbiome, nutrient deficiencies, hormonal imbalance, and toxicities. You are an individual, not a statistic. In functional medicine, your doctor has to work a bit harder—using the best data balanced against your individuality—to personalize your care.

The emerging complexities of individual health, combined with the inherent limitations of clinical trials, have even the most educated and respected medical experts expressing their doubts about clinical trials and what constitutes "evidence" in medicine. To start with, scientifically sound clinical trials have never been a prime mover of medical standards, nor do they always result in absolute answers. Way back in 1978, a report from the US Congressional Office of Technology Assessment concluded: "No more than 15% of medical interventions are supported by reliable scientific evidence." In 1991, Richard Smith, the editor of the *British Medical Journal*, commented that "only 1% of the articles in medical journals are scientifically sound—many treatments have not been assessed at all." And in 2009, Marcia Angell, former editor of the *New England Journal of Medicine*, wrote in the *New York Review of Books*:

It is simply no longer possible to believe much of the clinical research that is published, or to rely on the judgment of trusted physicians or authoritative medical guidelines. I take no pleasure in this conclusion, which I reached slowly and reluctantly over my two decades as an editor of the *New England Journal of Medicine.*

For those of us who entrust our lives, or our patients' lives, to the results of these studies, these conclusions can be a hard pill to swallow.

So what is it that makes clinical trials and research unreliable? First of all, clinical trials are designed with extremely narrow parameters for what constitutes success. If a clinical trial can demonstrate some effectiveness at treating singular symptoms in the people chosen for the study, then it is published as a success. A second issue is conflicts of interest: many clinical trials are sponsored by industries that stand to gain from the results, making unbiased reporting impossible even with the best intentions. Third, the time frames of the vast majority of clinical trials looking at vascular health are too short to reveal the long-term effects of a particular treatment or lifestyle. Clinical trials are expensive, so long-term trials are financially prohibitive. To compensate, many trials are of short duration, but conclude with a projection of what the researchers *think* will happen over time. This is why it took so long for the link between smoking and cancer to be revealed. Smoking for three years probably won't give you cancer. Smoking for thirty years will.

Finally, and perhaps most importantly, the complexity and ethics of experimentation on humans make it impossible to control for every factor in the interrelated network that makes up our complete health. Working for two years on a master's degree in a clinical trials center, it became obvious to me that even a trial run very ethically and with very high standards is not going to uncover the whole story about what is right for each individual. The hard part of working with you to develop your unique solution is that you, like every other person on the planet, are complicated and unique. But this is also why I work hard for my patients and why I've been inspired to write this book to show you how to heal your unique heart.

And now let's do just that. It is time to take everything you've learned in the previous chapters—and more importantly, everything you've learned from a lifetime of being the person who knows your body better than anyone—and build your own Precision, Personalized Solution to make your future the brightest and most vital it can be.

Precision, Personalized Assessment

To help you choose the lifestyle medicine that will benefit you the most, we need to determine where *you* stand on the spectrum of heart disease risk.

You and I can't interact here in the pages of this book in the same way we would if you came to my clinic, but the following assessment is designed to share with you the things I do in my clinic that you can do on your own, and give you the empowering experience of being both the patient and the expert. The Precision, Personalized Assessment contains four parts: (1) "The Heart Solution Matrix," (2) "Your Sources of Inflammation," (3) "Body Type," and (4) "Internal and External Clues." When you understand all four, your self-knowledge will be vast indeed. This knowledge will be the compass needle, pointing us toward a solution tailored specifically for you.

Consider this assessment to be a virtual walk into my clinic. Using what you learned about your body in the first part of this book and your vast experience being who you are, go through this assessment thinking about your pain points. Pain, fatigue, intestinal discomfort, brain fog, mood, and anxiety are the ways in which your body expresses dysfunction. These sensations are not just "in your head." They are real. But you can turn the table on your pain points by using them to your advantage—as clues to where your greatest opportunities to heal lie. Ask yourself the same question I'd be asking you if you were sitting in front of me in my clinic: What imbalance in your system is holding back your body's beautiful ability to heal and function optimally?

Please consider this assessment as honestly and completely as you can. At the end, the idea is not to have a final score, but rather a target for the lifestyle changes and nutrients that will benefit you most.

After you, the expert in the mirror, have completed the assessment, I'll give you my recommendations in Part III, "The Precision, Personalized Solution," on how to use lifestyle medicine to correct your particular imbalances—your prescription to yourself for lasting health and the reversal of heart disease. This will include nutrition advice, supplement recommendations, exercise strategies for a wide range of aerobic health levels, and guidance on working with your doctor to improve your heart health while minimizing your pharmaceutical use and maybe even reducing or eliminating any drugs you currently take.

The program I'm offering you in the next few pages is one you can undertake today without spending tons of money, taking drugs, or going to the doctor. But remember: ultimately, healing your heart is a continuum of care, and it starts with you.

1. The Heart Solution Matrix

The first step of your assessment is to complete the Heart Solution Matrix. It's similar to the Functional Medicine Matrix I use in my practice to determine which monsters may be sleeping (or roaring) in a patient's unique biology. When you're done, you'll be able to see the entirety of your complex heart health, and that perspective will give you insights into your own imbalances and where you need to focus your efforts at healing.

My operating assumption is that nearly everyone has imbalances and inflammation, and the goal here is to help you find your individual Achilles' heel—your pain points. What is it in your history, lifestyle, and unique biology that could make your heart function decline? When I see women work with conviction on repairing their pain points, their quality of life nearly always increases and their symptoms of dysfunction decrease or even disappear.

Family Health History

Do you have one or more family members who have suffered from (check all that apply):

☐ Heart disease

☐ Diabetes

☐ Obesity

☐ Alzheimer's disease or dementia

☐ Rheumatoid arthritis, lupus, or other autoimmune disease

☐ Crohn's disease, ulcerative colitis, or other inflammatory bowel disease

☐ Psoriasis or other serious skin disease

You've already learned that your genes are not your destiny. But sometimes reviewing our family history reminds us that we tend not only to have the same genes as our parents and grandparents but to eat similarly and lead similar lifestyles. If many of your family members have suffered from any of these ailments, shared lifestyles may be at least as much of a factor as genetics. We'll cover the many ways to adjust your own lifestyle for the better in Part III.

Personal Health History

Early life history

Consider your history starting from the very beginning. How were you born? A vaginal birth transfers crucial gut bacteria from mother to child that birth by cesarean section does not.

Did you have any childhood illnesses or take lots of antibiotics? Some of my patients reply to this question: "No, I didn't get antibiotics, but had my tonsils out and tubes in my ears twice." Well, this means they most certainly had lots of antibiotics, because a child has to undergo several rounds of antibiotics with no success before doctors resort to surgical procedures.

The worst scenario for the gut is having been born by c-section and having had your tonsils out. This combination wreaks havoc on the gut microbiome, dooming you to a life of fatigue, acne and other skin conditions, gut dysfunction, hormone imbalance, and eventually heart disease—unless, of course, you intentionally rebuild your microbiome, as I'll show you in Part III.

- **Nutritional deficiencies:** To help you consider the nutrients you may be deficient in, here are the top six nutritional deficiencies I see in my clinic, and the symptoms associated with them:

    - **Iron:** fatigue, weakness, bright red tongue

    - **Vitamin B12:** fatigue, numbness/tingling, mood issues, migraines

    - **Folate:** mood disorders, skin conditions, poor hair quality

    - **Vitamin D:** osteoporosis, autoimmune conditions, mood issues

    - **Zinc:** chronic infections, acne and other skin conditions, white spots on fingernails

- **Magnesium:** muscle twitching and cramps, constipation, irregular heartbeat

Along with potential deficiencies of specific nutrients, assess your body's big-picture nutrition by looking at the food you eat every day and considering how it may be contributing to nutritional deficiencies in your body. Do you eat:

- Large portions of simple carbohydrates—white flour, sugar, etc.

- A lot of low-quality protein—large fish (high in heavy metals), factory-farmed meat, heavily processed soy products

- Inadequate portions of low-quality vegetables and fruits— less than five cups daily of non-organic, low-variety fruits and vegetables

- Heavily processed, prepared food

- Sugary or high-carbohydrate drinks, including soda and juice

One of the most common deficiencies is usually accompanied by an excess: fat. Do you eat too much unhealthy fat and not enough healthy fat? I'll give you my complete and simple guide to fats in Chapter 6, but as part of your assessment, consider these symptoms of inadequate consumption of healthy fats:

- Low energy—feeling exhausted in the afternoon and resorting to naps, coffee, or sweets to make it through the day

- Cravings for carbohydrates like pizza, bread, and pasta

- Difficulty losing weight

- A feeling of lack of willpower when it comes to food choices

• **Food sensitivities:** Write down all of your known sensitivities. If you have not taken the food sensitivity test, consider doing a self-test by removing these three foods from your diet for thirty days. (I'll show you how in Part III.) This is the "Easy Three" that I see causing the most food sensitivities.

– Dairy

– Eggs

– Bread

Hormonal Imbalance

As you saw from Chapter 5, hormones are a crucial part of a woman's heart health, and two of the most critical components of hormonal balance are the thyroid and the adrenals.

Thyroid quiz

Let's start with a simple quiz for the most common signs of thyroid imbalance that we see in our clinic.

• Do you have unexplained fatigue and were you tested for thyroid function but told that your lab tests were "normal"?

• Have you been diagnosed with Hashimoto's thyroiditis or another thyroid disease?

• Do you have autoimmune disease?

• Do you have elevated cholesterol even though you eat optimally?

• Do you have difficulty losing weight or getting to your ideal weight?

• Do you have cold hands and feet?

• Are you dramatically more sensitive to the cold than you used to be?

- Are you experiencing hair loss, particularly thinning or brittle hair?

- Do you have dry skin?

- Do you sleep restlessly?

- Do you have low blood pressure or a low resting heart rate but do not engage in strenuous aerobic exercise and are not an athlete?

- Are you tired when you wake up even after a long night's sleep?

- Do you have depressed moods or just feel "flat" all the time?

- Is there a history of thyroid problems in your family, especially in the women in your family?

- Do you have an "afternoon lull"—fatigue and decreased energy between 2:00 and 4:00 p.m.?

- Do you experience undue difficulty concentrating?

If you answer yes to more than five of these questions, it's likely that you suffer from low thyroid function. You will want to focus on healing your thyroid in Part III (see page 290). You can also find supplements to support your thyroid on pages 290–294.

Adrenal quiz

And now a short quiz to see if you experience any of the most common symptoms of adrenal fatigue.

- Do you have unexplained fatigue but "normal" lab tests?

- Do you have airborne allergies or food sensitivities/intolerances?

- Do you have poor digestion, bloating, or irritable bowel syndrome?

- Do you have asthma, eczema, or irritations from chemicals?

- Do you have recurrent infections?

- Do you crave salt or sugar?

- Are you slow to recover from colds or flu or other illnesses?

- Are you slow to recover from injury?

- Have you been under severe emotional stress recently, or did you have severe life stressors in the last one to two years that left you not feeling "right"?

- Do you have low blood pressure and feel lightheaded when rising too quickly?

- Do you have depressed moods?

- Do you have anxiety/panic attacks, irritability, or impatience? Are you quick to get angry?

- Do you have low libido—low sexual drive or interest?

- Do you have hair loss, particularly fine thin hair with loss at the temples?

- Do you wake up in the middle of the night for no reason and find it difficult to fall back asleep?

- Does your energy fade in the afternoon?

- Do you feel tired most of the day, get a "second wind" in the evening, and then find it hard to fall asleep at night?

If you answered yes to more than five questions, you're likely to be suffering from adrenal fatigue/dysregulation. You can find Dr. Mark's Hormone Protocol on page 220.

The Hormone Disruptors in Your Environment

Reducing hormone disruptors is a crucial part of bolstering hormone health. See the sidebar on hormone disruptors (page 154) to get a better understanding of the ways in which they're infiltrating your home. Then mark all of the following items that you come in contact with on a regular basis.

1. **BPA**—Bisphenol A is released from many plastics when microwaved or heated and is present on cash register receipts. Also, recent research indicates that being "BPA free" doesn't necessarily mean the plastic is safer. Avoid heating plastics.

2. **Phthalates**—These chemicals are found in many plastics, over-the-counter medications, and in skin care, sunblock, and personal care products—especially those for kids!

3. **Fire retardants**—Your kid's brightly colored princess jammies and bedsheets are "fire retardant" thanks to chemicals that are known hormone disruptors—not what you want your daughter's thyroid and female hormones (or yours) sleeping in. Wash new clothes before wearing them.

4. **Lead**—Fortunately, lead was taken out of gasoline and paint, but it's been shown that lead will leach from the bones of older women who had more contact with lead (before regulation to reduce lead exposure). If you live in an older house that may have lead pipes (think Flint, Michigan), consider having your water tested.

5. **Arsenic**—Found in many Chinese over-the-counter supplements, arsenic also has been found in rice from some areas and shown to be much more common in rural water systems than ever imagined.

6. **Mercury**—You may already know that your silver fillings are only half silver and that the rest is mercury. You and your

dentist together can assess your risk. Also ask your doctor about preservative-free vaccines, which contain no mercury (marketed as thimerosol). The health effect of the low-bioavailability form of mercury used in vaccines is controversial, but when possible, I suggest not adding to your body's toxin load.

7. **Perfluorinated chemicals**—These chemicals are found in the Teflon coating on some cookware and in Scotchgard stain-proofing, Gore-Tex, and other coatings applied to upholstery and fabrics.

Hormone Disruptors

Hormone disruptors are chemicals that get into our bodies, find their way into the phone lines of our hormone communications, and cut the wires. This is why you should never microwave plastic. Heating plastic, especially in a microwave, can release bisphenol A (BPA), which is a known carcinogen and one of many chemicals that confuse your female hormones and can convert them from useful communicators to disease promoters. The problem is partially societal—as mentioned earlier, the average woman is exposed to 168 chemicals before she leaves the house, and several of these are hormone disruptors. Also, our food supply chain is full of hormone-laden food that gets into us and can cause this disruption.

It could also be your neighbor's fault! Medications are only partially used by the body before being excreted and ending up in the environment we all share. A researcher in Colorado, observing that the water downstream from Boulder contained

8. **Organophosphate pesticides**—These are the pesticides that have recently raised so much public concern over their use and overuse, especially in the malathion mosquito spray used in many communities. (I used to run behind the pesticide truck every summer, playing in the malathion fog being sprayed out behind it, as it drove through our neighborhood.)

9. **Glycol ethers**—These are in paints and stains, which should never be applied without respiratory protection. Also try to avoid the newly painted area for many days after application as it dries. Have an expert with proper safety equipment do

more synthetic hormones during the school year than during the summer, concluded that the birth control hormones taken by college students during the school year were passed through to the water supplies via their urine. And for now, municipal water filtration systems are not sophisticated enough to remove pharmaceuticals.

I turn to the Environmental Working Group for advice each year about the "Dirty Dozen" and the "Clean Fifteen"—the twelve most chemical-laden foods and the fifteen least toxic foods. Using these EWG rankings (www.ewg.org), I can recommend foods that have the fewest hormone-disrupting chemicals and are safest for optimal hormone production and communication. EWG also has a Skin Deep app (www.ewg.org/skindeep/app/) that rates most beauty products on a scale of 1 to 10 for toxicity. You really want to know what you—and the rest of your family—are putting on your skin!

the work while you go camping or to the beach for a week as the paint "cures" and becomes less volatile and less dangerous to you and your family!

Toxins and Toxic Exposures

As you learned in the last chapter, toxins are hidden drivers of heart problems, and removing dangerous toxins is a simple way to positively influence your health. Although the recommendation of one alcoholic drink per day for women and two for men is still widely touted as safe—and used as a rationalization for drinking— the studies behind that recommendation are now under scrutiny as new data emerge. The latest data indicates that even one drink a day may be doing more harm than good.

One study concluded that women over age fifty-five may be the only ones whose hearts benefit from (very light) alcohol consumption. (Finally, some heart health news that makes healing more fun for older women!) This means that if you're under fifty-five (or a man of any age) and think you're doing your heart a favor by sipping a glass or two of wine each night, you're probably kidding yourself.

On top of alcohol, we're subjected every day to the most toxic environment in human history. Our detox systems are pushed to the limit just dealing with unavoidable toxins. Don't add to your toxic burden. Consider these questions:

- How many alcoholic drinks do you have each week?

- How often do you smoke?

- How many chemicals do you apply to your body?

- Do you work or live in an industrial area?

- Is the water where you live tested for cleanness and high quality? (Ask your public works department for a copy of your water testing results.)

Your personal history is a great way to start thinking about the baseline of your overall health. Do you still need to heal from a significant number of past insults to your heart health? Did you run behind the mosquito sprayer like I did? Or grow up in an old house with lead paint? Do you think you may have adrenal or thyroid dysfunction? If you feel you have a lot of heart damage in your history, take Part III seriously and also consider enlisting a doctor qualified in hormonal medicine, detoxification, and nutrition to help you clean some of the skeletons out of your heart health closet and give you a fresh start.

Personal Lifestyle Factors

This is the part of the Precision, Personalized Assessment that we'd all love to just be able to pop a pill and avoid. Nobody likes taking a critical look at their own lifestyle. But as you go through this somewhat uncomfortable part of the assessment, please know that there is light at the end of the tunnel. Every one of the lifestyle factors that elevate your heart disease risk can be replaced by a lifestyle factor that reduces your risk and makes your life more enjoyable. Taking a critical look at the elements of your lifestyle that harm you is the first step to meeting the new you that is out there waiting to be discovered.

Food

- Do you consume fewer than five colored fruits and vegetables a day?

- Are you drinking less than half an ounce of water for every pound of your body weight (about six glasses for the average woman) each day?

- Do you regularly consume factory-farmed, supermarket-quality meat?

- Are you consuming meat over five times a week?

- Does your breakfast contain adequate fiber? (Sugary cereals that advertise their fiber content don't count.)

- Are simple carbohydrates the biggest portion of each of your meals?

- Have you ever fasted intermittently?

  When I ask if you've fasted, I don't mean the juice fast—drinking only juice for twenty-four to seventy-two hours, in my opinion, is not healthy—or a multi-day fast, but rather the intermittent fast of spacing your meals so as to have fifteen hours between dinner and breakfast the next day. (See Galen's fifth law on page 250 for specifics on the intermittent fast, and Chapter 6 on proper food.)

Rest

- Are you getting less than eight hours of sleep a night?

- Do you wake up tired?

- Do you have dreams (even if you can't remember what they are specifically)?

- Have you been diagnosed with sleep apnea?

- Do you have a partner who is a restless sleeper or who snores? Studies show that insomnia in women is often caused not by their own poor sleep, restless legs, snoring, or apnea, but by their partner's.

- Do you watch TV in bed before sleep or use your smart phone late at night?

  See Galen's third law on page 245 for sleep solutions.

Activities

- Do you get your heart rate up to a feeling of exertion fewer than three times per week?

- Do you do light exercise like yoga or stretching?

- Do you attempt more serious workouts like CrossFit or pilates?

- Do you spend more than two hours per day on the sofa?

- Do you spend more than six hours a day sitting down for work?

- Do you have to drive to work or to do your daily errands? If so, for how long?

- How much time do you spend on average on your feet each day?

  See Galen's second law on page 230 for my exercise solution.

Family and Friends

- Would you assess your relationship with your partner as below average?

- Do you have little or no social support from friends?

- Do you have fewer than two social engagements per week?

- Do you frequently have negative interactions with others?

- How frequently do you engage with family members?

Mood

- Do you enjoy your job?

- Do you have brain fog?

- Have you lost your "zest" for life? Are you excited about your day when you wake up?

- Do you find joy in your day from your relationships and family? Are your work and home life well balanced?

- Do you live in an unstable home or have an unstable relationship?

- Are you the primary caregiver for someone in your life?

- Do you frequently feel:

  - Angry (or, as my patients seem to prefer, "irritable")

  - Stressed out (wired and tired)

  - Overwhelmed to the point of inaction or poor choices

  - On the verge of tears in situations that didn't bring on tears in the past

  - Out of breath, chest tightness, tingling lips or fingers when anxious

  - Anxious over issues that didn't make you anxious in the past

  - Defeated or overly self-conscious in ways that cause inaction or poor choices

See Galen's sixth law on page 251 for recommendations on the benefits of social interaction.

Personal lifestyle factors can be the hardest to face, but take heart—even if you feel like your life is a smorgasbord of heart-damaging lifestyle factors, these are areas where great opportunity for healing can be found. They are the elements of heart health that are best optimized by you yourself, on your own time, without a doctor and without sacrificing too much of the lifestyle you enjoy.

2. Your Sources of Inflammation

After reading about inflammation in Chapter 3, you probably felt overwhelmed by just how many factors there are that contribute to inflammation, and therefore disease. From poor diet to lack of sleep to your morning commute, it's sometimes difficult to feel you have any control over your body.

The good news is that your body wants to heal. In fact, it is always trying to heal, even when it seems to be betraying you with debilitating and painful symptoms. The key is recognizing those areas of your life where you can do better—where you can help your body heal instead of making the problem worse. Before we dial in your Precision, Personalized Solution in Part III, it's important to take note of the places in your day where you let inflammation occur and the areas where you think you can improve.

My inflammation assessment is presented as a set of questions about the inflammatory insults you are likely to expose yourself to at different times of the day. This evaluation is based not only on confirmed science but also on my thirty-five years of experience helping people heal, one by one, by targeting and removing the inflammatory land mines they encounter in their lives. I offer specific anti-inflammatory strategies in Part III, but for now, consider the areas where you may be hiding inflammation.

Morning

- Do you wake up feeling refreshed?

- Do you fast for at least twelve and ideally fifteen hours between dinner and breakfast?

- Do you frequently forget or skip breakfast?

- Is the food you eat for breakfast low-quality and/or highly processed?

- Is your morning routine one of the most stressful parts of your day?

- Do you drink juice, soda, or several cups of low-quality coffee in the morning?

- Do you get any exercise by walking to work, walking your children to school, or going up a few flights of stairs in the morning? (Even light exercise will boost your metabolism and clear your mind for the day.)

Midday

- Do you skip a healthy snack in the late morning, but then find yourself reaching for the Danish or glazed doughnut left over from the work meeting?

- Do you pack your own lunch or "grab something quick"?

- Do you use saving money as a rationalization to eat fast food? (Fast food doesn't really save money.)

- Do you eat at your desk while working, or do you relax and enjoy your food?

- Do you feel indigestion or discomfort during or after lunch? (If so, change your breakfast.)

- On an average day, do you get exercise of any kind?

- Do you feel lonely during the day?

- Do you have sugar or coffee cravings in the afternoon to combat fatigue?

- Is your work or daytime routine stressful to the point of making you feel helpless or like "it's going to kill me"?

Evening

- Do you eat dinner late (after 8:00 p.m.)?

- Do you spend time socializing with your loved ones in the evening and at dinnertime, or do you all just do your own thing and eat as an afterthought?

- Do you feel bloated after dinner?

- Do you always eat a hefty portion of dessert?

- Do you frequently eat heavy desserts like ice cream and cake, or do you eat lighter desserts like sorbet and berries?

- Do you watch television more than about one hour a night on average?

- Do you often feel heartburn when you lie down?

- Is your sleep partner a big issue for the quality of your sleep?

We've all experienced the relief that follows a reduction of inflammation—like when a sprained ankle feels good enough to walk on again, a headache starts to fade, or final exams or the busy season at work finally pass. Once you have pinpointed one or two prime culprits causing your inflammation and addressed them with the solutions presented in Part III, you will feel that immense sense of relief as your systemic inflammation starts to decline—and will be that much more motivated to stick with your solution.

3. Body Type

The next—and simplest—part of this assessment is body type. When I see a new patient, her body type alone will give me much of the same information as blood tests or vital measurements like blood pressure and pulse. Body type is simple to assess, and one of the most revealing and scientifically valid windows into heart health.

In medical school, I was taught to use the ratio of height to weight to calculate body mass index (BMI). Well, what I've learned since then is that BMI is best suited as a tool for insurance companies to measure heart disease risk and calculate a financial premium accordingly—in other words, it's useless. As it turns out, the way the weight is distributed on the body is far more useful for determining an individual's imbalances and revealing internal function.

You may have heard of the "apple" or "pear" body type—two images that, as with so many body image issues, are most often used as descriptives for women's bodies. As a tool for assessing heart disease risk, body type is a telling assessment method for both women and men.

Being overweight doesn't feel good and reduces vitality, and obesity is a significant heart disease risk no matter where the weight is located, but when it comes to mapping your individual solution, these two body types carry different risks that are best treated through somewhat different solutions. If you don't fit either body type, stay tuned: there's a particular flavor of heart disease risk we sometimes call "skinny fat"—slender people who have energy pathway (metabolic) dysfunction.

The way to determine if you're the pear or apple body type is to find your waist-to-hip ratio (WHR). Recent data on the WHR show that the measurement is so important for diagnosing heart health that it should be considered a vital sign just like heart rate or temperature. In fact, WHR may be even more revealing of heart disease risk than many lab tests!

Determining Waist-to-Hip Ratio

Start with a long look in the mirror. Does your body seem to hold most of its fat in your midsection? That's the apple body type. Or does most of your body's fat ride lower on your hips and upper thighs? That's the pear body type. If you don't see any fat, good for you, but don't go away, you still may be in danger.

If you're unsure about your body type, get out a tape measure and measure your hips at the widest bony part where the upper leg bone and hip meet. This is your hip measurement.

Next feel your lowest rib and then, below it, the iliac crest of your pelvis, the bone at the very top of the hip. There are a few inches of space between that last rib and the pelvis on each side. Measure your waist circumference right between your lowest rib and the top of your iliac crest. This is your waist measurement.

Divide the waist measurement by the hip measurement to get the waist-to-hip ratio.

Your WHR is the easiest and most effective way for you to map your Precision, Personalized Solution because it gives you a place to start focusing your efforts that is supported by solid scientific data. It's an intimidating project to make real changes in your lifestyle with the hope that they'll improve your life enough to make the hassle worthwhile, and there are a multitude of ways to go about it, so you want to start with the changes that are likely to help you the most. Your WHR will give you a really good idea of where your troublemakers are found and what kind of therapies would give you the best bang for your buck when it comes to investing your energy and time in healing your heart.

As you read through the following guidance for different body types, remember that you may benefit from parts of the solution for a body type different from yours. For this reason, I suggest reading each one, but when you put down the book and set out to make real changes in life, start with the solutions presented as most applicable to your own body type.

The Apple Body Type

A waist-to-hip ratio greater than 0.85 for women (and greater than 1.0 for men) is a marker of the apple body type and an indicator of very high heart disease risk. A reader with this body type carries what we in the medical field call central obesity—visceral, hot, or internal fat. Body fat centered around the gut indicates a dramatically increased risk of heart disease. I tell my patients that none of us wants to carry fat on the outside of our bodies because we want to look good, but as the doctor who cares about you, it is the internal fat that concerns me the most.

The visceral fat that collects around the waist and inspires slang such as "muffin top" and "beer belly" is the most dangerous fat in the human body. This fat fuels the fires of inflammation. In people with this body shape, each of their organs is wrapped in a little (or not so little) cocoon of fat that provokes inflammatory messaging, interferes with hormonal communication, and wreaks such havoc in the body that some doctors look upon this visceral fat as functioning like a destructive organ of its own.

If you tend toward an apple-shaped body, as described by your WHR, you're likely to have dysfunction related to your metabolism (how you use energy), and your Precision, Personalized Solution should focus on:

Improving your energy use (metabolism): Reduce your sugar, processed foods, and simple carbohydrate consumption. Replace these calories with a rainbow of different-colored fruits and vegetables and satisfying but healthy fats, such as olive oil, high-quality meats, and other sources of protein.

Exercising daily: Exercise is the driver of metabolism. If you turn it up, your body warms up and releases hormones that tell your system to function more efficiently, with less inflammation, and to use calories rather than store them. See Chapter 7 for exercise recommendations across a wide range of fitness levels.

Consuming high-quality, nutrient-dense food: Stop buying packaged and prepared food. You want every calorie you eat to be used, not stored, because your particular body has learned to transform much of what you eat into the most damaging kind of fat your body can make.

Using the glycemic index in food choices: This will help you develop a sense of which foods will spike your blood sugar and add another layer of hot, toxic, visceral fat around your organs, and which foods will give you a nice sustained energy flow and allow you to process the sugar in your food at a pace that your insulin machine can handle without packing that sugar away as fat.

The Pear Body Type

A woman with a pear-shaped body—hips larger than the waist—tends to be at lower risk than a woman with an apple-shaped body for chronic inflammatory diseases like heart disease, diabetes, and Alzheimer's. But before you go have a celebratory scone, know that having a pear-shaped body doesn't mean you can eat whatever you want and leave exercise for the birds; it just means your system tends to store fat in a less inflammatory way than the apple body type does.

If you have a pear-shaped body, most likely the dysfunction in your heart and vascular system is information-related: some parts of the beautiful hormonal symphony of your thyroid, adrenal, and female hormones may be out of tune. If this is you, there's a good chance that some toxicity sprinkled over all of those hormones is making them less efficient and disrupting their communication.

Your Precision, Personalized Solution will benefit most from:

- Improving systemic communication by eliminating inflammatory triggers

- Optimizing thyroid function (see Chapter 8 on thyroid repair)

- Mitigating adrenal stress (see Galen's Six Other Laws in Chapter 7)

- Efficiently utilizing your female hormones (see Dr. Mark's Hormone Protocol in Chapter 6 and Chapter 8 for supplements by body type)

- Reducing your body's toxic burden

The Skinny Fat Body Type

Everyone loses muscle as they age, and the skinny fat body type is most common in people over fifty. But the skinny fat condition starts developing much earlier in life, usually among people who are not particularly active but can eat whatever they want without gaining weight. If this is you, you're probably the envy of all your friends, but beware: that natural tendency toward a slender figure can lead not only to less visible fat but also to less muscle and increased heart disease risk. Someone who struggles with weight gain and is constantly working hard to manage her waistline may very well be at lower risk for heart and brain disease than someone who keeps a slender figure no matter how much unhealthy fat and sugar she eats.

If you're naturally slender, the waist-to-hip ratio is not a valid way to assess your heart health. A better indicator is muscle mass relative to fat. Indicators that you may be skinny fat include:

- Elevated liver test (AST, ALT, GGT) showing a stressed liver

- High blood sugar or insulin

- Elevated blood pressure

- High triglycerides, low HDL cholesterol

- Low muscle mass compared to people of a similar weight

- Ability to consume lots of sugar and other carbs without gaining weight

- Carb craving

• Frequent fatigue with "brain fog"

• Any noticeable fat isolated to the belly

When it comes to heart health, muscle is your bank account. Muscle burns energy even when resting, heavily influences your metabolism, helps you eliminate toxins and reduce oxidative stress, and tells your systems to use nutrients rather than store them.

The problem with this body type is that not only are you missing the bank account of healthy muscle development, but the balance of your muscle mass to fat storage is very much a concern. I'm not talking about building up bulk, but rather maintaining a healthy skeletal musculature to see you through old age with function and health.

When we age, we not only lose muscle but it becomes more difficult to build more. A common condition among older thin women is sarcopenia, a degenerative loss of muscle. Frequently, this condition develops in conjunction with a small increase in belly fat that just never seems to go away. So if you are one of those "lucky" skinny fat women but are now noticing, as you approach middle age, a decline in muscle as well as a persistent but slight increase in fat stored around your belly, you may be more at risk for heart disease than you think.

A woman with the skinny fat body type has a particularly dangerous form of risk: doctors often do not target her as someone who needs further screening or therapy recommendations for heart health. If your doctor is one of those who still thinks heart disease isn't an issue for women, you can be sure that if you're skinny as well as a woman, heart disease will be the last thing on your doctor's mind. You should find another doctor.

If you suspect you are skinny fat, you'll want to study the recommendations for the pear and apple body types, because your imbalances are most likely both energy-related (like the apple body type) and inflammation- and hormone-related (like the pear body type). But with your skinny fat body type, you'll need to put a priority focus on the following three things:

- Build muscle

- Build muscle

- Build muscle

Yup, for the skinny fat body type, muscle is your heart's best friend. Muscle will be the driving factor in giving you a life that is not only long but full of health and vitality. If you have a skinny fat body type, your muscles are endangered, and if you lose muscle past a certain point, your doctor will diagnose you with sarcopenia, which has been linked to heart disease as well as Alzheimer's disease and is strongly linked to osteoporosis; sarcopenia patients have a much higher risk of hip fracture at a much younger age. The relationship between bone health, muscle structure, and heart disease is significant: studies show that over 30 percent of women who fracture a hip after the age of sixty-five die within one year!

If you've never been interested in exercise because you're naturally blessed with a slender figure, simply don't enjoy exertion, or do exercise but perhaps not in a way that builds muscle, read carefully when you get to the advice on exercise in Chapter 7. If you have fatigue issues, consider asking your doctor to test your blood sugar and liver function and to give you an advanced heart panel that includes cholesterol particle size and inflammation marker levels. (Chapter 9 will help you interpret these tests.) If you fit the skinny fat body type and have other elevated factors for heart disease risk, you should treat your solution with the same level of urgency as someone who is obese.

Healing and Your Body Type

The body type assessment may seem simplistic, but it is in fact an incredibly powerful assessment tool that is supported by research and commonly used by functional medicine physicians. It gives you a tangible and reliable picture of where you should put your efforts toward healing and also gives you a sense of your particular flavor of heart disease risk. See Chapter 8 for specific nutritional supplement recommendations for each body type.

Did you always have more of a pear-shaped body until menopause and now have enough of a little gut to be starting to identify with the apple shape? If so, your heart risk is rising quickly and you need to move fast to heal while you can.

Do you identify with the skinny fat body type? Figure out how to build muscle and put some deposits in your body's bank account.

Are you young and fit but can see the tendency to store fat around your waist? Adjust your lifestyle now and dial in your solution so you will have many more years of feeling young and fit.

Do you feel like you're hopelessly stuck with a body type that cannot change? Take hope. I see people of all ages change their body type through the Precision, Personalized Solution. It works because it's a program that is made for only one person: you. So let's take a closer look at you.

4. Internal and External Clues

The physical manifestations of heart health I am about to share with you are fascinating. Some stem from ancient medical theories that have recently been proven true by science, and some are subtle clues associated with different levels of heart disease risk and overall well-being. These observational assessment methods will not give you concrete answers, but my experience tells me that they will be extremely valuable as clues to help you decide where to focus your healing efforts.

The body loves to tell you its story. You just need to know how and where to listen for it.

Oral Clues

An emerging concern for heart disease lies in the mouth—your oral health speaks volumes about your heart health. Cavities, amalgams, extensive dental work, and gum disease can all be related to heart health.

For your evaluation in the mirror, consider your dental history and habits. Do you always brush and floss twice a day? If not, change your ways. Improving your oral health will also improve your heart health. Additionally, look at the texture and color of your tongue for clues to internal issues:

- Whiteness may suggest yeast overgrowth or gut bacterial imbalance.

- A patchy or "geographic" tongue that looks sort of like a map may indicate food sensitivities and nutritional deficiencies.

- Ridges on the side of the tongue may indicate low thyroid function.

- Small cracks on the side of the tongue or corner of the mouth may indicate vitamin B12 and other B vitamin deficiencies.

External Clues

Ruddy cheeks

Ruddiness in the cheeks can be an indication of internal inflammation and is a common characteristic of people admitted to the hospital for severe heart problems. Are your cheeks flushed all the time? If so, and if you identify with some of the other indicators of elevated heart disease risk in this book, you should consider consulting with a heart specialist with a holistic view of healing after you read Chapter 9 and learn how to work with your doctor.

Earlobe crease

Look at your earlobes. One of the most fascinating indicators of heart health is the earlobe crease. The ear crease sign is described in Chinese medicine texts on heart health dating back at least two thousand years. A crease in both earlobes is now proven to be correlated with increased risk of not just heart disease but sudden death from heart disease. (While you're examining your earlobes, remember that you're doing a two-thousand-year-old heart health assessment! How cool is that?)

Abnormal pupils

Next, look deeply into your eyes. Enlarged pupils even when the room is brightly lit suggest an overactive nervous system and confused adrenal glands, probably due to stress. Turn the light off and then back on again. If your pupils first reduce in size, as you would expect, but then expand again slightly, this is an indication that your adrenals are out of balance.

Arcus senilus

Another well-proven indicator of heart health in facial features is arcus senilus, a small blue circle surrounding the colored part of the center of the eye (the iris). This blue circle can be an indicator of abnormal cholesterol processing and overall elevated cholesterol levels. Abnormal copper levels can also cause a blue circle around the iris.

Dark skin areas

Look at the color of the skin under your eyes and on the back of your neck. Darkness under the eyes and on the back of the neck suggests blood sugar abnormalities and is common in individuals with diabetes. Look under your arms—dark areas under the armpits can be signs of blood sugar imbalances.

Buffalo hump

This not-very-nice term describes an abnormal fat deposition on the back of the neck that is likely to indicate serious sugar metabolism problems.

Skin tags

Small skin tags—little skin growths almost like little flappy warts—can be related to abnormal cholesterol metabolism, especially the bad fatty triglyceride parts, and are particularly a concern when seen around the eyes.

Skin bumps/Eczema

Look at your overall skin tone for abnormal patterns. Small little bumps on the backs of the arms are commonly related to food sensitivities, usually to dairy. Dermatologists use fancy names like *dermatitis papillaris* or *eczematous dermatitis* for these bumps and will usually prescribe some type of nasty steroid cream to beat them into submission. But these creams, like so many drugs, just soothe the symptom and don't fix the problem. When you remove inflammatory foods and heal your gut, these bumps tend to disappear.

Fingernails

Your fingernails give clues to your body's nutrient absorption and digestive function. White spots on the nails can indicate zinc deficiency and can also be caused by psoriasis or diabetes.

If your thumbnails tend to be flat and have ridges running across them at 90 degrees to the axis of your finger, it's an indication that you are probably not optimally utilizing nutrition, because of either poor nutritional intake or gut dysfunction that's causing poor nutrient absorption, particularly of B vitamins, including biotin.

Pitting of the nails, which looks like miniature craters in the nail, is usually a sign of overall nutritional deficiency, but it can also be a sign of psoriasis, an autoimmune skin disease that sometimes causes joint pain and arthritis. The pitting is also related to alopecia, a severe form of hair loss that is surprisingly common in women.

I see many women with dry, brittle, and fragile nails. This can be related to thyroid imbalance but usually indicates a deficiency of vitamin A, vitamin C, or the B vitamin biotin. The nails are so sensitive to nutrition that if you are hospitalized for a major illness, such as a heart attack, your fingernails and thumbnails will develop a large ridge that marks that seminal event, reflecting how poorly your body was functioning at that time in the nails' growth. As your health recovers and your body regains function and adequate nutrition, your nails stop forming the white lines as they grow out.

Another pattern of horizontal lines on your fingernails, known as Mees' lines, can be related to arsenic poisoning and are usually dark in color. Black spots under any one nail (there can be more than one) without any history of trauma to the nail warrant a trip to your doctor; I have seen several cases of melanoma under the fingernail missed by primary care doctors. (These telltale black spots can be found under toenails too).

Vaginal discomfort

If you have a vaginal discharge or burning and irritation in the vaginal area, you may be experiencing a flora imbalance or yeast overgrowth, and vaginal dryness would suggest a hormone imbalance. Anal itching or burning may indicate either digestive

Digestive Absorption: Not Just a Gut Problem

Look at the texture and pattern of your hair. Loss of hair on the temples or sides of the forehead suggests abnormal hormone balance. Brittle or broken hair strands, especially in the absence of new "baby" hair growth, suggests a problem with digestive absorption.

I have been amazed at how poor the digestive absorption is in my patients who have elevated heart disease risk. For some of them, we run advanced lab tests to examine the digestive enzymes and breakdown of fats and proteins, but usually I can find the answer with just a few questions, starting with this one: Do you wake up feeling bloated or do you feel bloated only after eating?

Most of my patients will think for a moment and then say, "I wake up feeling okay, and my belly is fine, but about an hour after a meal the bloat kicks in and stays there till I go to bed."

If this sounds familiar, you probably have digestive absorption issues and will benefit from taking a digestive enzyme with your meals. You don't necessarily need to take a vitamin or supplement—beneficial digestive enzymes can be found naturally in papaya and mango. All it takes is a single piece of tasty dried mango, but you do need to eat it with your meal for it be effective.

dysfunction or a yeast-bacteria imbalance, especially if your bowel movements are frequent, your stool is particularly foul-smelling, or mucus is left floating in the bowl. These indications of possibly undigested food parts in the bowel may be pointing to a lack of digestive enzymes.

Varicose veins and ankle swelling

How about your legs? If you have varicose veins, they may be due to genetics, but it's far more likely that they're caused by poor circulation and lack of movement over time. Is there swelling around your ankles when you take your socks off at night? This would suggest some stagnation in the lymphatic (drainage) systems of your body. If you have either of these conditions, moderate daily exercise is probably what you're missing most that could improve your overall health and decrease your heart disease risk.

Keeping External Clues in Perspective

The external clues of heart health are a mixed blessing: it's convenient to have a way to assess your own heart health without going to the doctor, but once you know what to look for, you can't stop seeing it everywhere. The next time you see someone with a ruddy complexion and an ear crease, you may not be able to resist considering the condition of their heart. Just keep in mind that while scientific studies have drawn connections between these indicators and heart health, that doesn't mean everyone who has these features has a bad heart. So don't ruin Thanksgiving dinner by pointing out everyone's heart risk features! But if you do have family members who seem to have some of these indicators of elevated heart disease risk, you might suggest that they borrow this book.

Internal Clues

After your external self-examination, it's time for an internal scan. You'll be able to do this scan much better than I could, even if you came to see me in my clinic, because nobody on earth knows how you feel better than you do.

How is your gut?

Most of the women I see in my clinic have had digestive issues their entire lives. Many have talked to doctors about the problem and been told "to just live with it" or "everyone has that," or they've been given the garbage-can diagnosis of "irritable bowel syndrome." I was told I had irritable bowel syndrome until age twenty, when I managed to resolve my issues myself.

In our clinic, irritable bowel syndrome does not exist after a patient's first visits. Yes, many women come in with this condition—they're constantly bloated and have either no bowel movements for several days or several, sometimes urgent, bowel movements per day. Sure, it can be caused by a parasite or other bug, but the majority of the time it is caused by inflammation of the gut due to the permeability of the intestines.

As we talked about earlier, if you have leaky gut, you probably have significant gut inflammation as well as heart and brain inflammation. Each woman who comes in with an irritable bowel syndrome diagnosis from another doctor has the condition for a unique reason. The next time you're hanging with your girlfriends, ask if they have had problems with their digestion. I wouldn't be surprised if nine of ten of them say yes, and most will tell you that, when they talked to their doctor about it, they were either ignored or told that they had the dreaded and unsolvable "irritable bowel" and they'd just have to live with it. So they did—feeling constantly bloated, having abnormal bowel patterns, and some even scheduling their lives around what their gut would decide to do that day.

Your goal is to get to the root cause of the irritation and inflammation—and fix it. In my clinic, we always succeed at reducing leaky gut and irritable bowel syndrome, and you can do it too. And once you know that your gut is no longer inflamed, you know that the fire in your heart now has a chance to cool down too.

So stay tuned—my full plan for healing leaky gut issues is just a few pages away.

How is your mood?

Women suffer from depression more than men. We know that for many people depression is really an inflammatory disorder. If the brain is on fire with inflammatory chemicals that slow down communication with the nerves, this inflammation can manifest as both depression and anxiety. If you have either depression or anxiety, your heart and brain are almost certainly inflamed. There are studies that clearly show that heart rhythms are different if you are depressed. And the heart rhythm values that accompany depression are associated with a dramatic increase in the risk of sudden death. In other words, depression changes your heart rhythm in ways that make you more vulnerable to dying of a heart attack. When the depression clears, the heart rhythm normalizes and the risk goes away.

And yes, even with zero risk factors for heart disease, you can die suddenly of a "broken heart" after a great personal loss. When I was a medical resident, a woman named Janet, a fifty-two-year-old marathon runner with no cholesterol issues or family history of heart disease, came into the ER after her husband was in a car accident. As she was taken back to the trauma room, her husband was shocked with the paddles of the defibrillator for the last time and pronounced dead right in front of her. After ten minutes, she became nauseous and started vomiting. The ER doctors all thought these were symptoms of a "grief reaction," which they did not consider significant or unusual.

When Janet couldn't stop vomiting for two hours, I wondered if it was her heart causing the problem, and so I ran an electro-cardiogram on her as a precaution. She had zero complaints of chest pain, but her electrocardiogram showed that she was in the middle of a massive heart attack. She was transferred to cardiac intensive care, and later that night this marathon runner with no heart disease risk factors died of a broken heart.

In my career, I have seen so many heart attacks in women that were confused with something else—abdominal pain, vertigo, dizziness, nonstop burping, chronic cough, vague joint pain, sweating in the absence of exertion, or sweating only when eating. In my experience, just about anything unusual can be a hidden sign of a heart attack in women.

Here are some questions for you to consider: Have you been di-agnosed with an anxiety condition? Are you on anti-anxiety med-ication? Are you deeply depressed? Have you ever been deeply depressed?

How are your relationships?

A good way to assess your own health is to look at the health of your partner and that of your social support group of friends. Women with healthy partners and friends tend to be healthier than those whose social circles are unhealthy. Sometimes the only way to remove that dysfunction from our lives is to make some difficult relationship decisions. If you feel you're lacking social support, try seeking out like-minded healthy friends to form a new social group. Whether through church, art activities, a dance class, a cooking class, a new sport, or a walking group, seek out those opportunities that are in every community to create this kind of support.

Loneliness may be one of the biggest risk factors for chronic disease, but some people find that improving their relationships is the hardest therapy recommended in this book. For others, however, healthy relationships form the backbone of their solution. If you have a supportive partner and friends, lean on them to help you realize your solution (and help them to realize their own).

Do you feel lonely? Do your friends tell you, "You're one of those people who never seems to need help, but if you do, I'm here to help?" (Hint: Let them help you.) How many times a week do you talk to your friends? Do you have a partner who can help you heal your heart?

ACE Score

The final piece of your assessment of your heart disease risk from internal cues is your ACE (Adverse Childhood Experiences) Score, which tells you something about your future health risk based on events that happened long ago. A seminal study was conducted in 1998 by Dr. Vincent Felitti, who was trying to understand why his obesity clinic patients found it so hard to sustain a healthy lifestyle. In his study, he used a questionnaire aimed at discerning any correlations between seven types of adverse early life experiences and health later in life. He found—as have many other researchers since then who used his ACE Score methodology—that people who score higher on this survey of past adverse experiences tend to have more health problems, including heart disease, depression, addiction, and liver disease as well as poor overall health.

Studies not only confirm what may seem instinctive—that events early in childhood would affect us much later in life—but also trace the effect of early trauma to an increased risk of many diseases as well as future hormonal and adrenal dysfunction. Combine this risk with some toxicity and nutrient deficiency and you have the perfect storm for heart disease. The correlation of traumatic childhood events with your future health is very strong, and I encourage all of you to take the quiz and calculate your ACE Score.

The most important thing to remember is that the ACE Score is only a guideline: if you experienced other types of toxic stress over months or years, those probably increased your risk of dire health consequences as well.

Prior to your eighteenth birthday:

Did a parent or other adult in the household often or very often . . . Swear at you, insult you, put you down, or humiliate you? Act in a way that made you afraid that you might be physically hurt?

No _____   Yes _____

If yes, enter 1 _____

Did a parent or other adult in the household often or very often . . . Push, grab, slap, or throw something at you? Hit you so hard that you had marks or were injured?

No _____   Yes _____

If yes, enter 1 _____

Did an adult or person at least five years older than you ever . . . Touch or fondle you or have you touch their body in a sexual way? Attempt or actually have oral, anal, or vaginal intercourse with you?

No _____   Yes _____

If yes, enter 1 _____

Did you often or very often feel that . . . No one in your family loved you or thought you were important or special? Your family didn't look out for each other, feel close to each other, or support each other?

No _____   Yes _____

If yes, enter 1 _____

Did you often or very often feel that . . . You didn't have enough to eat, had to wear dirty clothes, and had no one to protect you? Your parents were too drunk or high to take care of you or take you to the doctor if you needed it?

No _____   Yes _____

If yes, enter 1 _____

Were your parents ever separated or divorced?

No _____   Yes _____

If yes, enter 1 _____

Was your mother or stepmother sometimes, often, or very often . . . Pushed, grabbed, slapped, or had something thrown at her? Kicked, bitten, hit with a fist, or hit with something hard? Repeatedly hit for at least a few minutes or threatened with a gun or knife?

No _____   Yes _____

If yes, enter 1 _____

Did you live with anyone who was a problem drinker or alcoholic or who used street drugs?

No _____   Yes _____

If yes, enter 1 _____

Was a household member depressed or mentally ill, or did a household member attempt suicide?

No _____   Yes _____

If yes, enter 1 _____

Did a household member go to prison?

No _____   Yes _____

If yes, enter 1 _____

Now add up your "yes" answers: this is your ACE Score.

There is one point for each type of trauma. The higher your score, the higher your risk of current and future illness. If your score is higher than 4, some of your current problems are almost certainly related to your distant past, and you may want to seek out professional help to work on these issues. Sometimes this is the biggest breakthrough when it comes to protecting a woman's heart from future risk. I tell my patients to think of the ACE Score as a special type of cholesterol test that measures future heart risk brought on by childhood stress.

Coming Up: Your Precision, Personalized Solution

Now that you've identified the specific moments in your day when you may be triggering inflammation, confirmed your individual body type, tracked your specific symptoms and history, and assessed your internal and external clues for disease, you should have a better understanding of what parts of your system need the most help. These will be crucial factors as we move into your solution.

Before you read on, consider what you have learned about yourself in this assessment and then pick two or three things you want to work on. This is exactly what I do in my clinic after we complete a patient's assessment: I let her pick the problems she wants to solve. This strategy has two big benefits. First, my patient knows best what is ailing her, and second, because she chooses the problems to confront, she usually succeeds at solving them (and that, by the way, makes me look like a better doctor). Now it's your turn to do this. Take a deep breath. Even better, take a walk and think about your pain points. What imbalances do you want to solve?

You have already made great strides toward protecting your body from heart disease and reversing the symptoms you have by taking a look deep into who you are. It is this understanding that will drive the lifestyle choices that turn on your inner healer, which is more powerful and more capable than any doctor, drug, procedure, or program. As you read into Part III, keep in mind those two or three primary pain points or imbalances that you feel are doing you the most damage and prioritize the tools presented in the next section accordingly.

You don't need to fix everything at once. You can always go back and work on a different issue two months or even six months from now. That's exactly what we do in my clinic. Pick a problem. Solve it. Pick a problem. Solve it. Eventually there are no more problems to be solved, just maintenance. And believe me, solving your way to vitality is a beautiful thing.

Part III

The Precision, Personalized Solution

In the second century AD, a Greek doctor named Galen developed guidelines for health that were far ahead of his time. One of the most influential physicians in history, he is known as the "Surgeon to the Gladiators." He wrote five hundred essays about human health, outlining the benefits and pitfalls of lifestyle and food choices, and developed Galen's Seven Laws of Health:

1. Eat proper foods

2. Exercise

3. Get adequate sleep

4. Drink the right liquids

5. Have a daily bowel movement

6. Control your emotions

7. Breathe fresh air

When Galen wrote down these laws, almost two thousand years ago, he pretty much hit the nail on the head—so much so that if you follow his seven laws, you'll vastly improve your quality of life and prevent chronic disease more effectively than any pharmaceutical ever could. The hard part of keeping Galen's seven laws is following them nearly every day of your life.

In the next two chapters, I'll be using Galen's seven laws as an overarching guide, modernized from the functional medicine perspective and applicable to your primary goals for healing based on what you've learned about yourself.

So far you've learned about how your heart interacts with your brain, gut, and hormonal system and with the environment that surrounds and passes through your body. This is all fascinating, but how do you use that information to develop a plan to reduce your heart disease risk? There are many paths to this end, but the optimal path for you will be navigated best by the world's foremost expert in all things you: you. I want to stress that you are incredibly well prepared now for a life of health. You picked up this book, you read about the fundamentals of heart health, and you took the Precision, Personalized Assessment. You know your body type and your personal history, you've taken a long look inside yourself, and now it's time to get to the specifics. I couldn't be more excited to take you on this journey.

Chapter 6

Eat Proper Foods

Galen's first law, "eat proper foods," is first for a reason. There is nothing more important to the health of your heart and body than the right nutrition.

What Is "Proper Food" Anyway?

Proper food is food that has undergone few changes in its path from the soil, pasture, or sea to your plate. It's food in a state that is closest to the way food has been for millions of years—no heavy metal toxicity, no added hormones or antibiotics, no genetic modification, no chemical treatments like pesticides and coloring agents, and minimal processing.

As you know, I don't like the word "diet," so I use the most accurate term available for my proper food plan: personalized nutrition. As I mentioned already, the data suggest that the way the peoples of the Mediterranean eat may be more effective at preventing heart disease than any drug. Other cultures, such as the Japanese, have also given us clues as to what proper food can do for longevity and vitality. Applying these fundamentals of proper food to your personalized nutrition plan is the key. The thing I like about personalized nutrition is that it's easy to fit into your life, delicious, and varied. To heal your heart and optimize your life, follow these six proper food guidelines: eat minimally processed plants, clean protein, healthy fats, and nutritious flavorings; make food social; and avoid foods that cause sensitivities (and exercise a little every day).

Minimally Processed Plants

President Ronald Reagan had it wrong when he declared that ketchup should be considered a vegetable for kids' school lunches: ketchup is a condiment processed from tomatoes, with added sugar and salt—not a proper food. For heart health, minimally processed plants should make up the majority of what you eat. And remember that processing can begin before the plant is even a seed, with genetic modification. The plant may be further processed with pesticides and fertilizers as it grows, and then after the harvest it's often processed into derivatives of itself in factories where food products are built. Sure, some parts of processed food may be okay to eat, but since we know that much of it contributes to poor health, why eat it? Especially when proper food is so beneficial and readily available in our fortunate corner of the world?

The more we study the health ramifications of food consumption as well as the biochemistry of food sources, the better proper foods look. A big discussion in nutrition circles centers on phytonutrients, the chemicals in plants that give them their vibrant color, flavor, and protection from various insults, such as germs and bugs. When we consume plants, their phytonutrients become available to us. A surprising number of these phytochemicals have proven to be highly protective of the human heart and to reduce a wide range of diseases. Several have gained notoriety for being powerful medicine, including carotenoids, flavonoids, isoflavones, lycopene, resveratrol, and tocotrienols, to name a few of the 25,000 known phytonutrients. Phytonutrients have proven to be anti-inflammatory, antioxidative, antihypercholesterolemic (control elevated cholesterol levels), and anti-ischemic (sustain the blood supply, like aspirin), inhibit platelet aggregation (prevent clotting), and are even antiangiogenic (resist the development of tumor blood supplies).

If this sounds to you like plants are the ultimate heart medication, you're right. So powerful are their phytonutrients that research has concluded that these compounds should be models for future cardiovascular drug designs. You don't need to know the phytonutrient content of all fruits and vegetables. Instead, eating a rainbow of different-colored fruits and vegetables will give you all the phytonutrients you need. I suggest to my patients that they eat a minimum of six colors per day, which sounds like a lot but is pretty easy to do. Have a few carrots (get the organic multicolored ones!) with a sliced tomato and some greens and you are more than halfway there.

Supplement makers are pushing phytonutrient supplements, but before you take any, be sure to consult with a nutritionist or physician who is trained in supplement use. Some of these powerful compounds can have side effects when concentrated into supplement form. Also, like so many elements of optimal health, the best way to get what you need is from food, not a pill.

My favorite foods for phytonutrient concentrations are:

- Tomatoes

- Dark leafy greens

- Winter squash

- Cruciferous vegetables like broccoli and Brussels sprouts

- Soybeans (in non-GMO and minimally processed forms, like tofu or edamame)

- Red and purple berries

Another key aspect of proper food is that it should be organic—or close to it. Not long ago, all food was "organic." And only recently did we begin contaminating our food for the sake of production. In my opinion the non-organic food should have a special label and cost more to pay for the healthcare associated with producing and eating it. In any case, certified organic food is not just a higher-priced version of the same thing. Studies continue to show that organic fruits and vegetables contain more of the nutrients you need and fewer of the inflammatory elements that hurt you. Peer-reviewed literature notes that food grown organically contains significantly more vitamin C, iron, phosphorous, and magnesium, as well as lower amounts of certain heavy metals. Not only do organic foods have more of these critical nutrients, but their nutrients, minerals, and plant proteins are higher quality. Little useful research has studied the human health effects of consuming organic compared to non-organic foods, simply because the tests conducted so far have not been of long enough duration. Get this: the longest comparative study of the health effects of organic versus conventional foods lasted for two years—you'd be hard pressed to prove that smoking causes cancer with a study that lasted just two years.

And admit it, you can taste the difference. Your body knows. It's a rare conventional vegetable or fruit that tastes as delicious, has as luscious a texture, or is as satisfying to eat as an organic version of the same thing.

Clean Protein

Clean protein is proper food, and "clean" means the same thing with respect to animal and vegetable protein sources as "minimally processed" means for fruits and vegetables. The less processed and artificially manipulated the protein is, the better its amino acid and fat profile and the fewer unhealthy components it contains. There are fewer monosaturated fats in organic, grass-fed meat, as well as more omega-3 and less omega-6, and emerging evidence suggests that, while there is huge variability between species, there are nutritionally meaningful differences in composition between organic and conventional meats. This is why grass-fed or organic meats are healthier than factory-farmed meats treated with preservatives and flavorings, and why tofu is healthier than fake bacon derived from soy that is processed to taste vaguely like bacon (even quality real bacon is probably healthier for most people than fake bacon).

I recommend eating fish and poultry at least twice a week. Pasture-raised poultry is a good source of clean protein and an alternative way to get omega-3 fatty acids if you simply don't like fish. Avoid factory-raised fish as well as tuna, swordfish, and other top predators in favor of wild-caught fish with a low heavy metal content and the smaller, fatty fish listed in my guide to healthy fats in the next section. Fish raised in captivity are treated with pesticides and antibiotics to help them survive living in close quarters with other fish, so wild-caught fish is not only cleaner but, from the heart health perspective (remember how toxins and hormone disruptors fuel the fires of inflammation?), can make the difference between a food that is medicine and a food that is poison.

Limit red meat consumption to a couple of times per week, eat small portions, and be sure it is grass-fed, hormone- and antibiotic-free, and prepared with care—don't burn it, don't serve it with additional fat, and serve yourself a portion about the size of your palm.

Just as you can tell the difference between organic and conventional vegetables and fruits without looking at the label, your body knows which kind of animal protein is better. You can taste and feel the difference. Sure, a premium cut of factory-raised meat can taste pretty good, but the rich flavor and lower-fat texture of grass-fed meat is far superior.

For vegetarians, clean protein also means minimally processed protein sources. Soy products come in a dizzying array of flavors, shapes, and promises, but most of them are highly processed and are best consumed in small amounts or not at all. Most vegetarians probably eat too much soy; if you're a vegetarian and find yourself eating soy every day, consider these clean protein sources, and be sure they are organic:

- Quinoa, buckwheat, triticale, and amaranth (clean protein and a complex carb—all in one)

- Chia seeds

- Beans, lentils, spinach, peas, and artichokes

- Guava (the highest-protein fruit)

- Eggs (pasture-raised)

- Garbanzo beans (hummus)

- Nut butter

- Yogurt (grass-fed, sugar-free)

While protein choices are important, remember that, no matter what foods you choose, your body won't be able to utilize the protein if it is fighting the inflammation and chronic damage caused by food sensitivities.

Healthy Fats—The Dr. Mark Guide

Healthy fat is crucial for sustaining energy levels, heart function, healing, brain function, and hormone and cholesterol balance, for absorption of nutrients, vitamins, and minerals, for making food appetizing, and for satisfying the appetite; unhealthy fat is a knife to the heart—but the difference can be confusing. Consider this simple way to evaluate fats.

> **Mama's Monounsaturated:** Your mama would approve of the way these healthy fats treat your body. Olive and avocado oils are monounsaturated fats. Monounsaturated fats are typically liquid at room temperature, but many kinds solidify or partially solidify in the refrigerator. Consume as desired and choose organic, high-quality varieties. For heart health, replace other fats in your diet with organic monounsaturated fats.

Peculiar Polyunsaturated: Soybean, corn, cottonseed, and safflower oils are polyunsaturated fats and are typically liquid at room temperature and in the refrigerator. Omega-3 and omega-6 are polyunsaturated fats. Canola oil is a mixture of polyunsaturated and monosaturated. Think of polyunsaturated fats as peculiar because their impact on health depends on very specific qualities that are hard to assess standing in the grocery store or ordering off a menu. To err on the side of health, consume polyunsaturated fats in small amounts and only non-GMO, organic, high-quality varieties.

Sometimes Spectacular Saturated: These are the animal fats like butter and lard, as well as vegetable fats that tend to be solid at room temperature, like coconut oil. Because saturated fats can certainly damage your heart, they are only sometimes spectacular. To keep them spectacular, consume in low quantities and, like meat, only eat animal-derived saturated fats from clean (organic) sources.

Heinous Hydrogenated/Trans/Unsaturated Fats (the worst of the lot): These are polyunsaturated oils that have been heavily processed to make them solid at room temperature, such as margarine and the fats commonly found in cookies and baked goods with long shelf lives. You can create your own partially hydrogenated oil just by deep-frying something. These are so bad that the FDA recently removed trans fats status as "Generally Recognized as Safe." This means experts in laboratories and hospitals around the world agree: The heinous hydrogenated stuff is not safe to consume. So don't.

GOOD SOURCES OF FAT (ALL NEED TO BE ORGANIC)

- Coconut oil—unrefined, cold-pressed, virgin

- Extra-virgin olive oil—unfiltered, stored in a dark bottle in cool temperatures

- Tallow and bone broth—from grass-fed, organic beef and pork

- Seed oils—expeller- or cold-pressed

- Avocados and avocado oil

- Eggs—pasture-raised

- Oily fish—salmon, herring, sardines, mackerel, bluefish

- Butter—grass-fed, eaten in small portions

- Ghee—clarified butter from grass-fed sources

- Nuts, seeds, and seaweed—as alternative sources of omega-3

- Wakame seaweed is perhaps the best vegetarian source of omega-3: it has an incredible omega-3 to omega-6 ratio of 1:18.

To put my fat recommendations in a nutshell: Use more olive oil and less butter. Use organic canola or avocado oil for high heat. Avoid trans fats like margarine, most vegetable oils, and deep-fried foods. If you eat animal fats, consume only the highest-quality meat from organic, pasture-raised, grass-fed sources.

Use Nutritious Flavorings

Salt consumption is strongly associated with health problems in people with high blood pressure, diabetics, people over fifty years old, and African Americans. Our bodies do need sodium—the nutritional element of salt—but almost all of us eat way too much of it. In fact, 90 percent of Americans eat more than the recommended amount, and most of it comes from restaurant meals.

As you know by now, sugar is also problematic. Remember that women with diabetes have twice the risk of heart attack as men with diabetes (due to differences in hormones, body fat deposition and inflammatory response). As we discussed in Chapter 1, women's vascular systems are different from men's, and the effects of diabetes are no exception. The increase in blood pressure, decrease in good cholesterol, and increase in abdominal fat that accompany diabetes in both genders all are more pronounced in women. Dear reader, you really, really want to avoid high blood sugar levels.

To wean yourself off of both salt and sugar, try using more herbs and spices, many of which have nutrients and minerals that help your body heal from and resist disease. Some are so beneficial that we use them in supplement form as well as in food. A wonderful synergy happens when you replace salt and sugar with herbs and spices: the more flavorful result makes heart-healthy food taste better, so your palate adjusts to prefer healthier foods rather than salty or sugary processed foods.

The following four spices have particularly powerful health benefits and, when combined with a reduction in salt and sugar, will work wonders to help you heal your heart.

Cinnamon

In an unexpected use of a pumpkin pie ingredient, cinnamon as a supplement has been used against infection, migraines, and cramps, as well as to aid reproduction and regulate diabetics' insulin levels by fighting insulin resistance. Now research suggests that cinnamon may also reduce the risk of Alzheimer's disease. Compounds found in cinnamon have anti-inflammatory and antioxidant characteristics and have been shown to inhibit the dysfunction of a protein called tau. Tau protein is a normal part of healthy cell structures, particularly nerve fibers, but with oxidative damage, tau dysfunction causes the neurofibrillary tangles of Alzheimer's.

To test the effects of cinnamon in reducing insulin resistance and cognition, rats were fed a high-fat, high-sugar diet that led to insulin resistance and impaired cognition in middle age. Rats also fed cinnamon did not acquire insulin resistance and maintained better cognitive function in maze exercises than both the control group and the other sugar- and fat-fed rats. In humans, diabetics have lowered their blood sugar by as much as 29 percent by ingesting a quarter-teaspoon of cinnamon twice a day for forty days.

There is no downside to increasing your cinnamon consumption, and there may be significant benefit. Add it to your oatmeal breakfast and sprinkle it on fruit and yogurt for dessert, but remember that processed foods containing cinnamon usually include a pile of sugar and other carbohydrates, so get your cinnamon by adding it yourself, not by choosing the cinnamon Pop-Tarts. If you have, or are worried about metabolic syndrome (a combination of high blood pressure and blood sugar, dangerous cholesterol levels, and abdominal fat), consider taking cinnamon supplements as part of your treatment. The Ceylon version of cinnamon has demonstrated the most consistent benefit in lowering blood sugar.

Garlic

There is a good reason why garlic was one of the original medicines— ancient medical texts from Asia, Africa, and Europe all mention its health benefits. The earliest mention of garlic as a medicine is in the Codex Ebers, an Egyptian medical text over three thousand years old.

In modern times, clinical studies have shown that allicin is the chemical in garlic that gives it its healing properties. Allicin inhibits the enzymes involved in synthesizing fats, acts as an anti-clotting aid in preventing platelet aggregation, and reduces LDL (bad) cholesterol formation. A 1996 double-blind crossover study demonstrated that eating one clove of garlic daily lowers total cholesterol by almost 10 percent and raises HDL (good) cholesterol slightly. There are also theories that garlic lowers blood pressure and protects against oxidative stress.

As with many supplements, there are no long-term studies into the vascular protection offered by garlic. Some of the reports on it, however, are promising. Particularly relevant to heart disease prevention is garlic's apparent ability to increase the elastic qualities of blood vessels and increase blood flow to the smallest capillaries.

As with most foods, preparation is important to preserve garlic's protective qualities. Most importantly, overcooking garlic ruins its medicinal properties. This is one area where the legendary Mediterranean cooks have it wrong: don't put the garlic into hot olive oil at the beginning of the meal, but instead add the garlic at the end and cook it just enough to subdue and spread the flavor without browning it.

Ginger

A favorite as an old home-brewed, Depression-era cold medicine and remedy for gastrointestinal distress, ginger is another spice with incredible healing properties. Eaten regularly, ginger reduces inflammation thanks to potent anti-inflammatory compounds called gingerols. It has also proven effective at reducing nausea, and in at least one study it was more effective than Dramamine at reducing the symptoms of motion sickness. Clinical studies have demonstrated that individuals with rheumatoid arthritis and osteoarthritis who consume ginger regularly experience pain relief, decreased swelling, and increased mobility.

I know it seems far-fetched that the stuff we use to clean the palate between bites in the sushi restaurant can help prevent heart disease, but the data are clear: gingerol inhibits the production of nitric oxide, which contributes to the formation of inflammatory free radicals. This is why ginger is used prior to radiation therapy for cancer patients—to lessen the radiation's depletion of their bodies' antioxidant capacity.

Ginger is strong medicine, and no heart disease prevention refrigerator is complete without a ginger root in the crisper. Dried ginger powder retains some gingerol, but fresh ginger contains higher levels. It can also be frozen and will keep up to six months in the freezer. In the refrigerator, ginger should be stored with the peel on and consumed within three weeks.

Turmeric

Turmeric is the most powerful inflammation fighter in your spice cabinet, containing over two dozen anti-inflammatory compounds. The medical ingredient in turmeric is curcumin, which can be taken as a supplement. Curcumin works similar to Cox-2 inhibitors like ibuprofen: it blocks enzymes that cause inflammation. If you take curcumin as a supplement, make sure it's of nutraceutical quality with tested high absorption rates. You don't want to take curcumin made in an outdoor lab next to a coal-fired power plant in China. Piperine, a compound found in black pepper, is typically added to curcumin supplements to increase absorption; if you cook with turmeric, be sure to add a little black pepper to your recipe. There are now some very high-quality curcumin products on the market with potent anti-inflammatory effects.

Make Food Social

Dine with family and friends as much as possible. Why? Studies have shown that the risk of cardiovascular disease decreases as social support increases. Of course, many of the studies were done on men. However, research also suggests that social engagement may benefit women even more than men; as social engagement is reduced, health-related quality-of-life indicators drop much more significantly among women than men.

For this reason, I always include a prescription for socializing with my patients' solution. If you want to partake in the one alcoholic drink a day currently (but dubiously) recommended, go ahead, but drink it with someone you love. If you eat something you know will cause you intestinal grief, do so at a social event that is worth the recovery period you know you'll need afterwards. And when you prepare meals with proper food, share them with someone important to you so that you reap the rewards of proper nutrition along with social engagement.

The social aspect is one part of proper food that is all too often overlooked. Eating slowly, in a relaxed social atmosphere, is a key part of the health benefit of a personalized nutrition plan. No studies have proven it (yet), but I'm sure that proper food would show far less benefit ordered from a drive-through window and consumed while navigating rush-hour traffic, in the midst of a lonely life without social support.

Avoid Food Sensitivities

By now you are well aware of the powerful synergy that happens when you reduce the factors that cause a defensive reaction in your body: absorption of nutrients you do need is increased; your genes are bathed in a less inflammatory environment, which soothes the epigenetic expression of the inflammatory SNPs that may be lurking in your DNA; and your body's healing "bandwidth" is freed up to deal with other insults rather than constantly trying to heal from damage caused by its own defensive overreaction.

When one of my patients adjusts her nutrition plan to accommodate her food sensitivities, many of her pain points decrease in intensity or disappear altogether. These are some of my happiest patients because they aren't taking drugs, they didn't undergo expensive treatments, they can still eat delicious food, they're suffering from zero unpleasant side effects, and they now have a solution they can easily sustain for the rest of their lives.

As I mentioned during the Precision, Personalized Assessment, the three most common food sensitivities I see—and the easiest for you to experiment with—are the Easy Three: dairy, eggs, and bread. *If you have even the smallest suspicion that you may have food sensitivities, try going for one month without dairy, eggs, and bread—and if that's too much, try one at a time.* I suggest bread rather than gluten because bread products are easy get rid of, whereas you can drive yourself crazy trying to eliminate all the products containing gluten, like your toothpaste. From my clinical observation, the breads and gluten source that bother people the most are the "yeasty wheats." Some people may later need to try a super-strict gluten-free nutrition plan, yet most of the success I see in my clinic comes from eliminating one or more of the Easy Three.

Your main reasons for removing the Easy Three may be to lose those extra few pounds on your waist or to clear up your skin or to slow down the hair loss. But after just one month, you may find that not only are your main complaints better, but you are sleeping better and awakening more refreshed, your joints don't hurt so much at the end of the day, your mood is improved, your bowel movements are regular for the first time in years, and that belly bloating is gone.

After thirty days of avoiding the Easy Three, you then want to become a "food detective" (not the food police!). Slowly introduce one food from the Easy Three—one serving every few days—and monitor how you feel. Use the 7-Day Food Log (see appendix) to keep track of what you eat and also note your mood, energy, sleep quality, bloating, and bowel movements. As you fill in the log, you'll start to see your unique pattern.

When I eat something that I react to, the consequences are laughably predictable for my family and coworkers. I just love the everything bagel from the bakery two blocks down the street from my clinic, and sometimes I break down and get one when I drive by at 6:30 a.m., knowing that the bagels are fresh out of the oven and piping hot. The bagel tastes great, and I feel great (in the short term) as I spoil myself with a delicious treat. Around dinnertime, the bloating starts. My daughter, seeing my Buddha belly as we cook dinner, will say, "Dad, did you go for the everything bagel today?"

Yes, it is that noticeable. I also feel a little sluggish and brain-foggy by dinnertime if I eat a bagel in the morning. The worst part is then sleeping restlessly and waking up poorly rested and a little irritable, though the belly bloat will be gone. Then I'll go to work the day after eating the bagel and my staff, who know me well, will notice I'm grumpy and less energetic than normal and say, "Mark, did you do the everything bagel yesterday?" If I don't go back and get another everything time bomb, the bloat is gone by the end of the next day, but it takes twelve hours or so for the worst symptoms to arise, and forty-eight for them to dissipate.

Once you start tracking your foods, with or without the 7-Day Food Log, the patterns will become quite clear. Try these foods in place of the Easy Three:

Bread: Corn tortillas, yeast-free corn, quinoa, and baked goods using grains other than wheat

Dairy: Organic almond milk, soy milk, and rice milk of various flavors (look for the unsweetened versions)

Eggs: High-quality protein like wild game, fish, and nuts

If your experiments with the Easy Three don't reveal the root of your problems, ask your doctor for a food sensitivity test. In my opinion, this test should be as much a part of standard heart health screening as blood pressure and cholesterol tests. A $150 food sensitivity test will give you a huge head start and give you far more information than you can glean from experimentation.

The Dr. Mark Plate

The simplest food guideline I can recommend for resisting and reversing heart disease is the Dr. Mark Plate. It's not a food pyramid, it's not a diet, and it's not set in stone. The idea is to look at your food choices—whether you're ordering a restaurant meal, filling your shopping cart, or cooking at home—and strive for a breakdown of foods similar to what's shown in the graphic below.

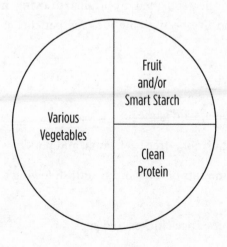

For fifteen years, the Dr. Mark Plate has been my go-to visual to encourage women get rid of the dirty word "diet" and develop a functional approach to personalized nutrition. Everyone benefits from this basic plan, a modified version of the Mediterranean diet. I originally created the Dr. Mark Plate for a mother of three with a full-time job and a stressed-out partner. She was overwhelmed with all the complex nutrition information out there and didn't know what to do. Preparing meals had become a terrible chore, full of fear that she was doing the wrong thing. So I pulled out a piece of paper, drew a sketch of the Dr. Mark Plate, and told her:

> When you think of a meal you are shopping for, preparing for your family, eating at a restaurant or at someone's house, fill your plate like this: half your plate should be multicolored vegetables, one-fourth of the plate should be protein, and for the last quarter a starch or carbohydrate and a piece of fruit, choose the ones that are whole-grain, gluten-free, and not significantly processed.

My patient breathed a sigh of relief—the Dr. Mark Plate was simple, tasty, varied, and easy for her to adapt to her busy life. After the idea worked so well for her, I adapted my original drawing into the graphic you see here, and I've been giving it to my patients as an easy food guide ever since.

CLEAN PROTEIN

Bison, venison, wild game

Grass-fed, hormone-free beef, lamb, and pork

Minimal amounts of tuna and swordfish (owing to mercury levels)

Organic, free-range chicken and eggs

Wild-caught fish (not farmed)

SMART STARCH

Quinoa

Wild rice and brown rice (avoid white rice)

Sweet potatoes and yams (avoid white potatoes)

FRUITS

Apples	Nectarines
Apricots	Oranges
Avocados	Papayas
Bananas	Peaches
Blackberries	Pears
Blueberries	Pineapples
Cherries	Plantains
Grapefruit	Plums
Grapes	Raspberries
Kiwis	Rhubarb
Lemons	Strawberries
Limes	Tangerines
Mangoes	Watermelon
Melons and cantaloupe	

VEGETABLES

Artichokes	Beets
Arugula	Bok choy
Asparagus	Broccoli and broccolini

Brussels sprouts

Cabbage

Carrots

Cauliflower

Celery

Cucumber

Eggplant

Garlic

Green beans

Green onions

Jicama

Kale

Kohlrabi

Lettuce

Onions

Parsley

Parsnip

Peppers

Radishes

Seaweed

Shallots

Snap peas

Spinach

Squash

Sweet potatoes

Tomatillos

Tomatoes

Turnips

GOOD FATS AND OILS

Avocado oil

Coconut oil

Extra-virgin olive oil

Grass-fed butter

Macadamia oil

NUTS AND SEEDS

Almonds

Brazil nuts

Hazelnuts

Macadamia nuts

Pecans

Pine nuts

Pistachios   Sunflower seeds

Pumpkin seeds   Walnuts

BEVERAGES

Almond milk   Filtered water

Coconut milk   Herbal tea

Coconut water   Mineral water

SUPERFOODS

Fermented foods (sauerkraut, fermented vegetables, kefir, kombucha)

Homemade bone broth

Organic unsweetened Greek yogurt

A Day of Proper Food

In Chapter 3, we covered what not to do when we followed an inflammatory day through the eyes and vascular system of a woman named Claire. So what should you do instead? The answer depends, of course, on the individual. To help you find the best food choices for yourself, I'll start with some general guidelines that I give to all my patients, then go through a day with recommendations for each meal as well as while traveling and on special occasions such as holidays.

There are a million reasons why we end up unable to follow a nutrition plan, and that can be okay. If you find yourself eating food you are unsure of, one of the best ways to gauge its inflammatory effect on your body is to assess how you feel at your next meal. Are you hungrier than usual? Are you shaky, as though you have low blood sugar? Do you feel bloated? If so, the previous meal was probably an inflammatory influence. If you have sustained energy, are comfortably satisfied, and feeling hungry but not starving after a reasonable interval, then your previous meal was probably a good choice.

Consider the following options for heart-healthy food choices at different times of day and in different scenarios. Of course, your food sensitivities, palate, shopping options, budget, and interest in cooking will affect your choices, but this is a good place to start to see what anti-inflammatory, balanced nutrition looks like over the course of a day. Please also see the glycemic index information later in this chapter.

Breakfast

This is where it all starts. If you're ever wondering how to eat at any point during the day, remember this: *Eat breakfast like a queen, lunch like a princess, and dinner like a pauper.* In other words, start your day with a proper meal, eat well at lunch, and eat a simple dinner.

If you are not sensitive to eggs, they are a great breakfast food, but only eat hormone-free, organic, pasture-raised eggs. Most breakfast meats are loaded with preservatives, and organic versions are very expensive.

Whenever my patients feel overwhelmed with food choices, I give them a simple breakfast plan that has worked for thousands of women: make a milkshake, and not any old milkshake but a delicious, healthy, clean, digestible, anti-inflammatory protein smoothie. The following Dr. Mark recipe for morning success can fuel most women, with even blood sugar, from as early as 6:00 a.m. until at least 1:00 p.m.

Protein Smoothie

10 ounces of organic coconut milk (spend the extra $1.50 per carton on organic)

1 scoop of clean, organic, pea-based protein smoothie mix (**www. menoclinic.com/smoothies**)

1 organic banana (you can use any fruit really—blueberries
work great)

1 tablespoon of organic peanut butter or almond butter

A few pieces of ice

Mix this all together in a blender (I like the handy bullet-type
blender) and in one minute you have a healthy, organic
inexpensive breakfast!

Look for organic fruit on sale and buy extra to store in the freezer, including berries, fresh fruit from the farmers' market, and bananas (peel before freezing). Freezing fruit saves time and money, and makes the smoothie cool and creamy. In my clinic staff room, we have a blender and protein powder and make smoothies daily, both for ourselves and to share with our patients as we show them how to make their own. And on occasion we have a smoothie dance party in the office!

Bircher muesli

The Swiss physician Maximilian Bircher-Benner developed
this simple breakfast for his patients around 1900. There are
a hundred variations, but start by mixing raw rolled oats and
chopped or ground nuts with your milk-like liquid of choice.
I suggest organic almond or oat milk, fruit juice (because of
the fiber in the oats and the small quantity of juice, this is a
healthy way to use fruit juice), or just water. Cover and soak
the mixture overnight in the refrigerator. In the morning, add
fresh fruit and yogurt, mix, and enjoy.

An oat-based breakfast is high on my list of ways to add
complex carbohydrates as well as fiber to your day. Oats
provide an excellent opportunity to personalize your

nutrition plan to fit your taste and lifestyle. The key here is to figure out what is best and most appealing for you, not just follow a recipe.

The better you are to your gut and yourself on a daily basis, the better the decisions you'll make about food choices, and here's why: after you eat twenty healthy breakfasts in a row, then eat eggs Benedict and a Danish with a glass of orange juice, you'll feel so much worse than you did the previous twenty days that you'll wait forty days before indulging again. *Eating proper food tunes your body to notice the damage of eating poorly.*

Lunch

Modern women are multitaskers, multiple hat–wearers, workers, super-moms, students, and care providers (maybe you're all of the above!), and lunch can all too easily slip into junk food haste. Find the time, even a few minutes, to relax and enjoy lunch. Remember that your desk (or couch) is not a table for eating at. No matter how short your lunch moment may be, sit down away from your work, take off your many hats, and use that midday meal as a chance to nurture yourself.

The key to an easy, healthy, inexpensive lunch starts with dinner the night before. Make a little extra protein for dinner, then bring this leftover to work in a glass (not plastic) container and add it to a salad of organic greens, avocados, small organic tomatoes, multicolored carrots, a little feta cheese, and a simple olive oil and balsamic vinegar dressing. And remember that protein doesn't have to be meat; seasoned and baked tofu, quinoa, legumes, or beans are great choices.

It's easy to make the mistake of thinking that a high-quality organic lunch is too expensive for everyday nutrition. Well, do the math for a week of salad:

$5 for organic greens

$3 for organic tomatoes

$3 for two organic avocados

$3 for olive oil dressing

$4 for clean feta cheese

$10 for clean protein

This comes out to $5.60 per day for high-quality, organic, pasture-raised, hormone-free lunches. Try it! You'll feel great, and it is the easiest lunch in the world once you get into the routine. (And if you factor in the reduced vitality and health care costs associated with junk food, proper food is the least expensive choice of all.)

Dinner

So often in the evening, after a cortisol-loaded day full of challenges, you're standing in your kitchen wondering what to cook. Or you're going out with family or friends to share a meal—maybe even finally going to that restaurant you've always wanted to share with your favorite person.

There's no need to deny yourself or feel punished, but in general do make this meal your cleanest and lightest for optimal body weight, deep sleep, and reduced overall inflammation—all of which add up to lower heart risk! The secret to a healthy dinner is sharing it. Have you heard the advice about never going to bed angry at your partner? Well, I feel it is even more important to not eat dinner alone. The social aspect of the evening dinner table is a lost art in society, with families increasingly unlikely to sit down and dine together, and reviving it is something I recommend to all of my patients.

From a proper food perspective, dinner is the time to catch up on any nutrition you may have missed throughout the day, and to slow down and think about what your body really needs. Didn't eat enough vegetables at breakfast and lunch? Make a nice big Niçoise salad with brown rice, fish, and a rainbow of multicolored vegetables with olive oil and your favorite spices. Craving fats? Add a side of avocado and drizzle olive oil over your meal. Feeling like your gut could use some probiotic help? Add a side of fermented food like sauerkraut or kimchi and have a cup of kefir and berries for desert (see fermented foods section coming up).

You've probably had that experience of a fatty fast-food meal late at night that just doesn't sit well and ruins your beauty sleep—this is your body telling you that what you ate wasn't a good choice. Think of dinner as the meal that sets you up for a good night's sleep, and the source of leftovers that will ensure you have an easy heart-healing lunch in your bag when you leave for work the next day.

Snacks and Eating While Traveling

Food choices while traveling can be unappealing at best and, at worst, downright horrifying. The key to thriving while crossing the proper-food deserts of travel is to carry a little of your proper food medicine cabinet with you. Put a small bag of nuts and dried fruit (the original breakfast), a piece of durable fresh fruit (such as an orange), and a high-quality protein bar (with minimal ingredients) in your purse to keep yourself from indulging in nasty snacks along the way. If you find yourself without your proper food stash, buy food that is closest to its natural form—for example, popcorn (without fake butter) is better than corn chips.

Granola with unsweetened organic Greek yogurt and fruit may be the healthiest and most readily available travel breakfast option. You'll see this breakfast offered even at the airport Starbucks. Of course, Starbucks also offers a croissant or muffin sandwich with not-so-clean ham and cheese. Choose the yogurt and fruit instead.

One of the greatest inventions in recent years for health-minded travelers is the foil pouches containing nut butters. Slip a few into your purse, and when proper food is scarce, spread it on slices of apple, a banana, or other fruit. This combination is a great choice because it satisfies both fat and sugar cravings and the blend of the carbohydrate, protein, and fats in the nut butter, combined with the fiber and not-too-much sugar of the fruit, makes for an ideal energy source. Just know that not all nut butters are created equal. During World War II, jars of peanut butter were air-dropped in North Africa to feed starving people. Some of those jars continue to be found today, and owing to the hydrogenated fat and preservative additives, the peanut butter is still just as edible as it was in 1940! Read labels. Try to find one with no sugar or other additives.

For your on-the-road dinner plans, the key is to have that morning protein and a healthy snack to calm the midday hangrys so that you don't roll into dinner ready to binge like a Roman. When you're contemplating a restaurant menu, remember that those terribly appealing fat-soaked and high–glycemic index meals will only taste and feel good for the first few bites. Thinking about ordering cordon bleu? You know those first bites are heaven, but the last bites feel like you're force-feeding yourself like a goose doomed to the fois gras industry. What about the grilled lemon herb chicken salad? You'll enjoy every bite equally, feel great afterwards, sleep better than if you'd chosen the cordon bleu, and feel more energetic the next morning because your body didn't spend half the night processing saturated and trans fats.

Also, try to eat early when you can—this gives you more opportunity to find a restaurant with healthier options, and sets up your internal cycle for healing. In the next chapter, we talk about intermittent fasting: having dinner at 6:00 p.m. and then waiting to have the morning meal or smoothie at 9:00 a.m. Daily fasting helps to optimize weight management and keep inflammation and blood sugar in check. Even if you can only pull off the fifteen-hour fast a few nights a week, it will help minimize the damage from the stress of travel.

Holidays and Special Occasions

Now we are getting to the heavy lifting. Combine typically rich food with sauces and gravies, extra meats with alcohol and sugary desserts, and you have the recipe for disaster. Now don't get me wrong, holiday food can be a wonderful and healthy passion, as long as it doesn't become poison. These are the meals that you must be most careful to keep from sabotaging all of your hard work. Have you ever had that huge Thanksgiving meal that sends you to the couch for the rest of the day feeling like the Goodyear blimp? Most of us have, even though we know, from eating the same meal the year before, that it's going to take a week to fully recover from it. I call this food amnesia—you forget how miserable it felt last year, so you do it all over again.

It's commonly said that the average American gains five pounds during the holidays, but it's not quite that bad. Studies have shown that we tend to gain about a pound over the holidays. The bad part is that we don't lose it over the rest of the year. So over a decade, we can blame ten pounds of fat storage on the holidays. It doesn't have to be that way. To minimize the holiday damage:

> Exercise on the holiday itself to increase your metabolism and burn more of what you eat rather than store it.
>
> Prepare at least one heart-healthy (and delicious) main course so you have something to enjoy that is also good for you.
>
> Go into the event agreeing with yourself to have one-half of whatever you think you want and think about the Dr. Mark Plate as you serve yourself.
>
> Have a heart-healthy breakfast that morning so you go into the holiday meal with stable blood sugar.
>
> Volunteer to be the designated driver. Excess alcohol is one of the more damaging parts of the holiday tradition.
>
> Most of all, enjoy those great meals. They are usually shared with the people you love, and social medicine is better than anything I can prescribe.

Calories and Food

Like Meredith, my patient who had tried every diet she came across before coming to my clinic for a kaleidoscope of serious issues, many women are told, "Calories in, calories out. If you are not losing weight, it is your fault for eating too much and not exercising enough." When I ask my patients if they've heard this before, they almost always nod their heads and say, "Yes, that is what I was told."

Then I say, "You probably believed it and did that exactly—ate less and exercised more and nothing happened, so you got mad at yourself and blamed yourself and gave up, right?"

They usually tell me that's almost exactly what happened.

I then tell them that this idea that calories in equals calories out is a myth. When researchers take the bacteria out of the gut of a skinny mouse and put it into an obese mouse and both mice consume the same diet, guess what happens? The obese mouse loses weight. It is the microbiome activity of the skinny mouse's transplanted bacteria that helps the obese mouse lose weight, not the calories consumed versus the calories burned. The microbiome can extract different amounts of calories from the same food, so if your gut is out of balance, you will never lose weight by cutting calories.

Everything we have been taught about counting calories is wrong. Every week women come into my clinic and tell me that they heard that a 1,000-calorie diet is a good way to lose weight. Well, not if the 1,000 calories are from a bagel with cream cheese, a cinnamon roll, and a large orange juice. On the other end of the spectrum, a piece of chicken, two vegetables, and a piece of fruit may also have 1,000 calories, but your body's metabolism will respond very differently to those calories. *Choose foods based on the nutrition in the food, the glycemic index, and your knowledge of how your body reacts to that nutrition, not the number of calories.*

Weight Loss, Hormones, and Diabetes

Considering the glycemic index in your personalized nutrition plan is essential because metabolic (energy) dysfunction is the root cause of diabetes, weight gain, and hormone imbalance. Insulin problems are greatly exacerbated by consumption of high-glycemic foods that contribute to the damaging condition called insulin sensitivity: the cellular equivalent of someone who keeps knocking on your door trying to sell you something you don't want or need until eventually you stop opening the door. What happens is that high blood sugars from processed and high-glycemic foods cause the insulin to keep knocking on the cells' doors to let sugar in even when the cells don't need the sugar—and eventually the cells ignore the knock. Then your pancreas does what it's supposed to do when there's too much sugar in the bloodstream: it increases insulin production to handle all the sugar. Since your cells don't need the sugar, the insulin takes the sugar to your liver which packages it up and stores it as that hot internal visceral fat that is so dangerous for the heart.

I wish I could tell you the dysfunction stops there, but no such luck. The increased insulin talks to your body fat and produces message interrupters that confuse your hormones and contribute to mood issues, PMS difficulties, menopause symptoms, infertility, fatigue, brain fog, sleep problems, skin conditions, and joint pain—and sets you on the path toward heart disease. If you already have heart disease, this process is that much more dangerous because your system is already seriously compromised.

The bright side of the interconnectedness of the body's system is that every positive action you take toward optimizing your health has a synergistically positive support reaction. When you choose low-glycemic foods with nice flat blood sugar curves to reduce your blood sugar and diabetes risk, you also lose weight, avoid the hormone-disrupting insulin dump of high blood sugar spikes, and your body stores less fat. You prevent the development of a diabetes or diabetes-like state and reap the rewards of a smorgasbord of benefits: you burn fat that may be stored in your body already, balance hormone levels, sleep better, improve your mood, find PMS and menopause easier, grow more energetic and sharper of mind, avoid premature infertility, heal from skin conditions and joint pain—and resist and even reverse heart disease.

The key to turning this cascade of damage into a synergy of healing is to focus on your metabolism. We are all still hardwired like our an-

Glycemic Index Comparison

High-Glycemic Foods

Angel food cake

Bagels

Brown rice pasta

Candy

Carrots

Corn chips

Corn flakes

Croissant

Doughnuts

Dried fruit

English muffins

French baguettes

French fries

Fruit juice

Graham crackers

High-fiber crisp

   rye bread

Honey

Macaroni and

   cheese

Pineapple

Popcorn

Puffed wheat

   cereal

Pumpkin

Raisins

Rice cakes

Rye flour

Semolina

Shortbread

Shredded wheat

Soft drinks

Tofu frozen

   dessert

Waffles

Watermelon

Wheat bran

White potatoes

Moderate-Glycemic Foods

Baked beans

Bananas

Blueberries

Buckwheat

Chocolate

Corn

Fruit cocktail,

   canned without

   added sugar

Green peas

Kiwifruit

Linguine

Macaroni

Mango

Noodles, instant

Pizza, cheese

Potato chips

Romano beans

Spaghetti, durum

Sweet potatoes

Yams

Low-Glycemic Foods

Apples

Apricots

Barley

Black beans

Blackberries

Black-eyed peas

Butter beans

Celery

Cherries

Chickpeas

Grapes

Grapefruit

Green beans

Kidney beans

Leafy greens

Lentils

Lima beans

Mushrooms

Navy beans

Oranges

Peaches

Pears

Peppers

Plums

Raspberries

Rice bran

Rye

Soybeans

Spaghetti, whole

   wheat

Strawberries

cestors, who probably started their day with a breakfast of nuts, fiber, and meat. Like us, they would have needed a good protein source in the morning to sustain energy through the rest of the day. Such a breakfast will not only bolster your energy levels throughout the day but train your body to harvest energy from your fat stores rather than store unusable sugars. And as you'll see in my hormone protocol, the entire messaging system of your body will benefit.

The Dr. Mark Hormone Protocol

This four-step prescription for balancing your hormones through food and lifestyle choices has formed the core of the solution for hundreds of my patients with dozens of different symptoms and diagnoses. Remember when I promised a way to address thyroid/adrenal imbalance and tune your symphony? This is it!

1. **Achieve optimal nutrition**

   - **Cut out dairy, gluten, sugar, and excess alcohol:** These are the foods that drive inflammation in the body and wreak havoc on your hormones (and cause problems for your skin).

   - **Replace poor-quality calories with greens, clean protein, and healthy fat:** These foods will give you the ideal balance of nutrients, antioxidants, fatty acid cellular building blocks, and protein fuel to balance your hormones (and keep your skin healthy).

   - **Choose optimal meats:** If you like seafood, reduce your consumption of red meat by replacing it with wild-caught fish, which are full of the anti-inflammatory omega-3 fatty acids. Try to avoid all factory-farmed animals and buy pasture-raised, grass-fed meats to reduce the antibiotics and hormones in your body.

   - **Figure out your personal food sensitivities:** To reduce hormone-disrupting inflammation in your body, identify the adrenal-depleting, thyroid-confusing, skin-damaging, inflammatory foods your body is reactive to or intolerant of.

2. **Support your gut microbiome to control inflammation**

- Use probiotic supplements to support an optimal anti-inflammatory balance and keep your skin clear.

- Eliminate anti-inflammatory medicines such as ibuprofen, which may disrupt this microbiome and make the gut permeable and inflamed, leading to hormone imbalance.

- Increase your intake of probiotics as well as prebiotics, the food that the probiotics eat. You don't need a pill for this. Try sauerkraut, kimchi, pickled vegetables, artichokes, dandelion greens, onion, leeks, and asparagus.

- You need to move your bowels daily. Ayurvedic medicine, the three-thousand-year-old health wisdom from India (even older than Galen's Seven Laws of Health), emphasizes having a bowel movement every morning to clear the toxins from the day before. The keys to doing this are adequate fiber (from the fruit-and-vegetable section of the grocery store, not the fiber wafers from the pharmacy section!), water, and probiotics.

3. **Use supplements to support hormone balance (see list below), but do not undergo hormone therapy without physician supervision**

- I recommend a professional-grade, plant-based protein smoothie (such as the recipe provided in "A Day of Proper Food"), which provides a clean and optimal protein start to the day but can be used at any meal. One of my weight loss secrets is to have a protein smoothie each meal for one week as a cleanse. Doing this seems to cool off the inflammation causing the hormonal, adrenal, and thyroid confusion that can throw the symphony out of harmony. Heal the gut, and the hormones follow.

- If you suspect hormone imbalance or disruption, consider the following supplements (see Chapter 8 for specifics on dosage and food sources of these hormone-healing supplements):

  – Vitamin D3/K2

  – Curcumin

  – Probiotic

  – Diindolemethane (DIM)

  – Magnesium

4. **Daily fasting**
   Daily fasting (spacing dinner and breakfast as much as 16 hours apart) is associated with decreased inflammation, strengthening of the immune system, optimized metabolism and hormone balance (see Chapter 7).

5. **Calm your mind so your body will behave**

- Chronic stress depletes cortisol over time, instigating a "cortisol steal" where your female hormones are effectively stolen by your stress response in order to produce adrenal hormones. So it's important to find a stress management technique that works for you. Exercise is excellent stress reduction, and consider using an app like Headspace or Muse for guided meditations. If an orchestrated meditation is too time-consuming for your life, try meditating for brief periods of time—at a stoplight, at the dinner table, before bed after a busy day—as described in Chapter 7. Additionally, the blood sugar spikes that drive the insulin response also cause cortisol problems, so optimal nutrition focused on low-glycemic foods is important for hormonal health.

Healing Leaky Gut

We're all well-trained consumers who like to buy something, do something, or add something in order to solve any problem, but the first stage of healing the gut is to *remove* a few things from your life. Do your best to eliminate, or at least reduce, the following primary culprits that damage the critical, doubles-tennis-court-wide-but-one-cell-thin, endothelial layer that lines your intestines:

- Pain medications (see Chapter 9 for natural replacements for pain meds)

- Processed foods (you know what to do—eat proper foods)

- Excess sugar (not only the obvious sources, like soda, but the hidden ones, like pasta sauce)

- Foods that trigger food sensitivities or intolerances (invest in a food sensitivity test but avoid the online tests, which offer a hair test they promise is just as reliable as a blood test—it's not)

- Chronic stress (see Chapter 7)

- Gut infections

- Poor sleep (see Chapter 7)

- Antibiotics (see Chapter 8 on how to avoid antibiotics or, if you must take them, repair the damage they cause)

Reducing or eliminating these stressors might just heal your gut even if you do nothing else, but here are the things you can add to your life to help heal your gut.

Eat Fermented Foods Every Day

Fermented foods include sauerkraut, kombucha (no sugar added), kimchi, kefir, kvass, and raw milk yogurt. Remember, pickles are preserved through the action of the acidity of vinegar, which is different from the fermenting process. So even though pickles may seem close to fermented on the flavor spectrum, they will do nothing to heal your gut and bolster the health of your microbiome. The Japanese ferment a wide range of vegetables, which may partly explain their legendary health, but we don't have as many fermented options in America. To eat more fermented foods, try these tricks:

- Add sauerkraut to sandwiches.

- Add kimchi (a spicy Korean-style fermented cabbage available in most grocery stores) as a condiment to almost every kind of dinner meal.

- Eat unsweetened yogurt with fruit for dessert (unless you have severe dairy sensitivities).

- Look for fermented vegetables in Asian specialty stores and order them at sushi restaurants.

Drink Bone Broth

Bone broth has become all the rage in some health circles, for good reason. It is rich in collagen, the superhero amino acid glutamine, glucosamine, magnesium, calcium, and more—all in a form that is easy for your body to absorb and utilize. The best bone broth is homemade. If you toss the bones after carving the meat off, you are throwing powerful medicine in the trash.

Instead, save the bones after a meal or even freeze them for later use. When you're ready to make broth, simmer the bones with a splash of vinegar (to extract nutrients) in a slow cooker for at least eight hours, and as long as thirty-six hours. If you're rushed, you can simply simmer them on the stove for a couple of hours, but you won't harvest as much of the bones' goodness as you will with the longer cooking time. When finished simmering, remove the bones, strain the liquid to remove the smaller bone fragments, and use the resulting broth for soup stock, or drink it hot right off the stove! Chicken and turkey carcasses, shanks, T-bones and ribs—all are fair game for bone broth. Once you start making bone broth from your leftover bones, you'll never waste them again. At quality meat counters, you can also buy hormone-free, grass-fed bones, which are quite inexpensive because most people think bones are for the dog.

Support Digestion

Remember the debate about whether heartburn is caused by too much or too little stomach acid? Well, we want to get it just right, and we know that digestion isn't a process isolated to the stomach. It also is driven by the brain. If you're stressed, exhausted, in a hurry, or otherwise out of balance emotionally, you won't digest nutrients as well. This is why it's so hard to step out of a stressful situation and immediately dig in to a big meal. Take the following steps to encourage proper digestion:

- Before eating, take a few deep belly breaths (see "Breathing for Healing" on page 252).

- Chew your food thoroughly so that it's sufficiently broken down and mixed with saliva before you swallow.

- Avoid drinking water or other liquids with your meals. I know it sounds unpleasant, but you do get used to it quickly.

- Before a protein-rich meal, drink one to two teaspoons of apple cider vinegar.

- If your doctor says you have low levels of stomach acid, consider using HCL (hydrochloric acid) supplements before your meal.

- Determine your food sensitivities and eat accordingly. (See Chapter 9 for food sensitivity testing guidelines.)

- Eat a slice of dried papaya or mango with meals—these foods contain an enzyme called papain that aids in digestion (it's the same stuff used in meat tenderizers).

Lectins and Autoimmunity

Lectins are sugar-binding proteins that are abundant in raw legumes and grains, and most commonly found in parts of seeds that become the leaves when the plant sprouts. Lectin proteins are resistant to human digestion and enter the blood unchanged.

Our bodies produce antibodies to lectins because we don't digest them, and nearly everyone has antibodies to some dietary lectins in their body. However, the response by each individual may vary, and the various lectins may have different consequences. The current concern is that for some select individuals, these lectin proteins drive leaky gut and inflammation.

In my clinical experience, just like dairy and wheat, the lectins are a problem for some people but not everyone. I suggest only trying to eliminate lectins if you're struggling with autoimmune disease or have intestinal issues and have tried everything else without success. Testing is evolving for this inflammatory protein and currently is not ready for prime time.

The Foundation of Vitality

We know a lot about nutrition, but, in my opinion, we have much to learn. The relationships between nutrition, the microbiome of organisms in your gut, and epigenetic expression are ripe for breakthrough medicine. But what's even more exciting is that all of these can be manipulated by you in what you choose to eat today. In an incredible example of gut health, a study in Japan showed that germ-free (no microbiome) mice release twice the amount of stress hormone when subjected to distressful situations as normal mice.

The relationships between the gut and the brain are so profound that a new field of study has emerged to research them: psychobiotics. If the gut is influencing the brain so profoundly, it is certainly driving heart health as well. One nutrition factor alone, inadequate fiber, can weaken gut bacteria known to be associated with resisting both depression and heart disease. Add metabolism, blood sugar, fat storage, energy, vascular health, hormonal messaging, and immune response to the equation, and nothing in your being is free from the impacts of nutrition, good or bad. Proper food is the link between all the elements of the Precision, Personalized Solution and the foundation of all disease resistance and vitality.

Chapter 7

The Other Six Laws

Now that you've learned what to eat and how to benefit from fueling your life and healing with proper food, you'll find even more benefit from this chapter's modernized functional medicine guide to Galen's six other two-thousand-year-old laws for healing the heart (and everything else). Here is a refresher:

GALEN'S SEVEN LAWS OF HEALTH

1. Eat proper foods (we just covered this!)

2. Exercise

3. Get adequate sleep

4. Drink the right liquids

5. Have a daily bowel movement

6. Control your emotions

7. Breathe fresh air

Law #2: Exercise

When it comes to exercise, as with many other things, we're a society of extremes. Here in Jackson Hole we have an unofficial event, called "the Picnic," that illustrates one extreme. It's done mostly by mountain fanatics who wake up at 4:00 a.m., bike 25 miles from the town square to Jenny Lake at the base of the Tetons, swim three miles across the freezing cold lake, climb 7,000 vertical feet to the summit of the Grand Teton, and then climb back down, swim back across the lake, bike back to town, and have pizza dinner with their friends by 9:00 p.m.

Culturally, our idea of exercise is out of whack—many of us get either too much or too little. Being a binge exerciser is better than doing nothing, but moderate exercise almost every day is far better for healing and avoiding heart disease.

Exercise increases oxidative stress in the body, but frequent exercise builds your body's natural ability to reduce oxidative stress; in other words, exercise can be both an oxidant and an antioxidant. Some oxidative stress is a good thing. It bolsters your cells' ability to handle the oxidation that happens when our muscles convert nutrients to energy. The stress causes you to build stronger muscles, and these muscles make you stronger not only in your external interactions with the world but also in your internal world—where metabolism and detoxification help manage oxidative stress, hormonal balance, brain function, and heart health.

One problem in our culture is that we associate exercise with sport more than health. Starting in elementary school, we go to gym class—where we learn sports. Sure, we get exercise in PE, and the class helps us endure sitting at desks the rest of the day, but we don't learn that frequent aerobic exercise is at least as important for a functional human being as math, reading, and the rest of the school curriculum. Even health class covers exercise in only the most rudimentary fashion (and often isn't even taught anymore because of the increased demands of standardized academic testing).

One of the greatest challenges for women (and men) trying to exercise is their employers, who typically foster sedentary working environments that provide little opportunity for movement. These employers don't realize that facilitating regular exercise will make for more productive, healthier, and better employees. Articles in business publications ranging from the *Harvard Business Review* to *Forbes* have trumpeted the compelling data clearly showing that paying staff to exercise regularly pays dividends. Progressive companies are figuring it out and installing gyms and climbing walls and encouraging regular exercise breaks to improve learning, concentration, creativity, mood, stress management, and memory. *And regular, moderately strenuous aerobic exercise is also the most powerful medicine of all for keeping you from suffering from heart disease.*

We're now deep into the Precision, Personalized Solution for heart health, and aerobic exercise is a crucial part of it. The great thing about pursuing heart health is that many prevention strategies increase the overall quality of your life. Exercise can so easily be adapted to your particular interests. Are you a night owl and like to dance? Great, take yourself dancing several nights a week! One of the first American mountaineers to climb K2, the world's second-highest mountain, trained by going out dancing every night all winter long—and he was the fittest climber on the mountain that year. If you can avoid the cocktails that too often go with a night of dancing, why not make dancing your exercise medicine?

Are you a morning person? Make a habit of greeting the sunrise during a brisk walk. Prefer staying inside? Get a stationary bike or a gym membership. Afraid of exercise? Start by just going for a walk. Park your car a little farther from the store. Walk down the hall to talk to a colleague rather than send an email.

Because It Feels Good

For millennia, the idea of going to exercise was absurd—everyday life was strenuous enough. If some people in the elite social classes managed

Brain Muscle

Exercise, when not pursued to excess, improves virtually every system in your body. We've known for a long time that exercise is a crucial element of any heart maintenance or repair program, but emerging evidence shows that exercise protects and helps repair not only our hearts but also our brains. For instance, research has uncovered several connections between Alzheimer's and exercise:

- Biomarker (measurable substance) studies of brain scans have revealed that individuals with greater "at-risk" indicators for Alzheimer's also tend to be sedentary, and that individuals who exercise have lower at-risk indicators.

- Exercise is particularly beneficial in reducing and delaying cognitive decline in individuals with a genetic predisposition for Alzheimer's.

- In as little as eighteen months, the hippocampus of the brains of people diagnosed with Alzheimer's shows a

to avoid exercise, few lived long enough for it to catch up to them. Even today, those of us who exercise so we'll live longer, disease-free lives are constantly explaining ourselves or putting up with comments like:

"What are you training for?"

"You're skinny enough already."

"Take the night off, you work too hard."

"Are you getting ready for the Tour de France or something?"

measurable 3 percent shrinkage—unless they exercise, and then there is almost no shrinkage.

- Alzheimer's victims who exercise have less accumulation of beta-amyloid plaques and tau tangles of the neurons—Alzheimer's telltale signs.

In a study at the University of Maryland School of Public Health, exercise was used as a treatment for cognitive decline. Individuals with mild cognitive impairment used exercise in conjunction with memory tests. MRI tests revealed that the exercise program significantly increased the intensity of their brain activity—including in the areas of the brain where Alzheimer's disease is diagnosed. Dr. J. Carson Smith concluded:

We found that after 12 weeks of being on a moderate exercise program, study participants improved their neural efficiency—basically they were using fewer neural resources to perform the same memory task. *No study has shown that a drug can do what we showed is possible with exercise.*

It's easy to feel it's not enough just to get your heart rate up—that you're expected to dress the part, buy the gear, and cop the whole persona of an athlete. You don't have to. The next time someone makes one of these comments when you're heading out or coming back from a hike, bike ride, or jog, remind them of this scene from the film *The Fisher King*: the character played by Robin Williams rubs his naked bum on the grass in New York's Central Park and says, "Do you know why dogs do this? Because it feels good!"

The first step in making exercise part of your Precision, Personalized Solution is to not let the hype of sport bother you. It doesn't matter if you're an "athlete" or not. Once you get into regular exercise, the benefits of living in a fitter, sexier, happier, younger-feeling body are so rewarding that you won't care what other people think.

Exercise was the original therapy,
and it may still be the most important.

Exercise has been integral in all practices of medicine, from Galen's Seven Laws of Health to the vast modern and historical library of research on the connection between exercise and heart health. Exercise is one thing, I'm proud to say, that medicine got right from the very beginning.

But exercise as a critical part of daily life hasn't become part of our culture in the same way that other health standards have. Most parents make their kids brush their teeth every day and wash their hands before eating to avoid disease, but how many parents make sure their kids get aerobic activity every day? As a culture, we need to treat exercise as a necessary part of daily life, not as just recreation. Since we're not there yet, you'll have to set this standard for yourself.

How Is the Aerobic Health of Your Heart?

Even though we've known for a long time that exercise is good for health, it's taken time for the methods of using exercise as medicine to evolve. It wasn't until 1963 that a cardiologist named Robert Bruce developed what became known as the Bruce Protocol Treadmill Stress Test, a way of using what was then new technology—the treadmill and the electrocardiogram—to determine an individual's baseline fitness and cardiovascular health. Before the Bruce Protocol, doctors assessed people either at rest or without a standardized comparison method.

A key component of the Bruce Protocol is the Metabolic Equivalency of Task (MET): a comparison of the energy burned while active compared to the resting metabolic rate. Many exercise machines and treadmills in your local gym or spa show MET levels on their digital displays to tell you how much energy you're burning by doing the exercise. One MET is one kilocalorie per kilogram per hour, or approximately the energy you burn while lying still doing absolutely nothing. For comparison, here are some approximated MET levels reached while participating in these different activities for one hour:

Lying still—1

Watching sports—1.5

Answering emails—1.8

Walking slowly—2

Showering and getting
    dressed—2.1

Automobile repair—2.93

Cleaning your house—3.01

Yoga—3.1

Playing with your kids—3.3

Walking briskly—3.3

Gardening and lawn
    work—3.66

Golfing—3.75

Fishing and hunting—4.5

Making love—5.0

Hiking—6.0

Skiing—7.0

Running—7.5

Cycling and basketball—8.0

Mountaineering—9.5

Martial arts—10.0

Running at a full sprint—15

Rowing or Nordic
    skiing—18

Several factors could, of course, change these estimates. Any of these activities done at varying intensities will burn more or less energy, and if you're skilled at an activity you can do it with less energy exertion. But thinking about MET levels gives you a way to monitor the health of your internal energy machine, which runs only as well as your heart does. Remember that the MET is a relative score comparing the energy expended on an activity to at-rest energy use. So a minute of martial arts uses ten times the energy of a minute of rest, and ten minutes of martial arts uses ten times more energy than ten minutes of rest. Cardiovascular fitness is directly related to the kind of MET output your body is capable of reaching and for how long. The MET increases with time spent doing a particular activity. Running fast up a hill burns about 8 MET in the first minute. Consider these generalized maximum MET levels for people of different fitness levels:

Post–heart attack patient—3 MET

Average but healthy person—10–12 MET

Person with above-average health—15 MET

Elite athlete—18 MET

This means that cleaning the house, even for one minute, would push the cardiovascular limits of many post–heart attack patients. Your personal MET, which gives you an idea of whether your heart and brain are receiving adequate oxygen, has profound implications for your heart health. Studies have shown that for each single MET increase, you reduce your chances of stroke, heart attack, and sudden death by 12.5 percent. If you increase your MET by four points—going from a fitness level that can handle fishing to being able to play basketball—you'll essentially reduce your chance of heart attack by half.

Self-Designed Exercise

Without visiting a functional medicine or similar holistically minded physician or finding a personal trainer who understands exercise for heart health rather than sport, how do you know how much exercise is enough? Debate on this point is undecided and controversial, and the recommendations vary widely. It would be great if everyone knew what it feels like to exert at 80 percent of maximum heart rate, but unfortunately the modern lifestyle does not encourage familiarity with exercise. Coming to know the sensations of aerobic activity is an important part of your Precision, Personalized Solution. The following section offers recommendations for developing an exercise plan to those who are unfamiliar with these sensations, at high risk for heart disease, or new to cardiovascular exertion.

My research has led me to two recommendations: one for maintaining overall cardiovascular health and one for a slightly higher level of exertion that will lower blood pressure and cholesterol (and *heal* the heart). To maintain cardiovascular health, engage in moderate activity for thirty minutes five days a week and in muscle-strengthening activity of moderate to high intensity two days a week. This is enough exercise to prevent weight gain and reduce the risk of many chronic diseases. To heal your heart, try to work toward forty-five minutes of moderate to vigorous aerobic activity five or six times a week, with a couple of days that also include muscle-strengthening activities. Your target heart rate for ideal cardiovascular benefit is 60 to 80 percent of your maximum. (I'll show you how to calculate this in a moment.)

That said, these recommendations mean very different things for different people. The bottom line is that you must find a way to fit exercise into your life on a nearly daily basis. For my patients who are intimidated by the very idea of exercise, I tell them to just start walking a little, every day.

You'll notice that my exercise recommendations almost never include rest days. That's because I know you're likely to take a day or two of rest each week anyway, either by choice or because life has a way of changing even the best-laid plans. The emerging evidence on vascular disease reversal, including experimental Alzheimer's disease treatments, is that six days a week of exercise is optimal for healing vascular damage in both the heart and the brain.

It's possible to assess your own fitness level with incredible accuracy but it takes raising your heart rate to a relatively high level. If you feel that your fitness is exceptionally poor, if you find that even light exercise causes symptoms like a head rush and heavy breathing, or if after even mild exertion it seems to take forever for your heart rate to slow down, it may be best to hire a trainer or get a doctor to advise you on the best fitness program.

I believe that anyone can reduce their heart disease risk by increasing their exercise level slowly and continuously over time. In the following section, I'll share my recommendations on exercise for the vast range of patients I see in my clinic.

Determining Your Fitness Level

The most revealing reflection of your heart health is your heart rate recovery, which you can calculate with a simple three-step test. First you determine your maximum heart rate based on your age, then you exercise until your heart rate reaches 80 percent of this maximum, and finally you calculate how much your heart rate slows down after one minute of rest. *The more quickly your heart slows down after exertion, the better your heart health.*

But before you get out the stopwatch and jump on the treadmill, I'm thinking you already have a pretty good idea of where you stand on the spectrum of aerobic health. After you walk up a few flights of stairs, does your heart feel like it's racing for a couple of minutes? Or do you feel your heart slowing noticeably as you walk down the hall from the top of the stairs? Do you get winded loading groceries into the car or does your pulse hardly change? Do you feel like your heart is dramatically weaker than when you were a teenager, or just about as strong? I'm going to explain how the heart rate recovery test works, but if you're truthful with yourself, you already know much of what you need to know to assess your heart health.

Maximum heart rate is an approximate safe upper limit for an average person of your age. The maximum heart rate of an elite marathon runner will be significantly higher than the recommended maximum for a woman who had a heart attack six months earlier. In other words, your heart health may not be perfectly assessed by this equation, but unless you're at one of the two ends of the aerobic health spectrum, it will give you a good idea of your optimal heart rate for heart-beneficial exercise.

If you get easily winded, are obese, or find even small amounts of exercise uncomfortable, consult with a personal trainer before doing this test.

The standard maximum heart rate calculation is 220 minus your age. For the heart rate recovery test, you want to elevate your heart rate to 80 percent of this maximum. So, for example, the maximum heart rate equation for a forty-year-old would be: $(220 - 40) * 80\% = 144$. Her target heart rate to test recovery is 144 beats per minute.

To determine her heart rate recovery, this forty-year-old will:

1. Increase her heart rate to 144 beats per minute by walking fast, running, getting on the stationary bike, or doing anything that pumps up her heart rate and allows her to check it often.

2. Continue exercising at that level for one minute.

3. Stop and check her heart rate. She'll do this by counting her pulse not for a full minute but for fifteen seconds, then multiplying by four. This method more accurately measures the heart rate at the moment she stopped exercising.

4. Rest for one minute, then check her pulse again.

5. Determine her heart rate recovery by calculating the difference between her heart rate when she stopped exercising and her heart rate one minute later.

A heart rate monitor simplifies this process, and I recommend buying or borrowing one to determine your baseline—or, better yet, test your heart rate recovery at a health club with a trainer to help. However you do it, the bottom line is this: *the faster you recover, the healthier your heart.* The bigger the difference between the two measurements of your heart rate the better; you want your heart to slow down significantly after only one minute of rest.

The difference between a strong heart that recovers quickly and a weak heart that takes a long time to recover is so dramatic that scientists use the terms "biological age" and "chronological age" to explain the difference. Essentially, if your heart recovers quickly, it is biologically *younger* than your chronological age would suggest. This is a good thing. If your heart recovers slowly, it is *older* than your chronological age would suggest. Not what you want.

If the difference between your heart rate when you stopped the exertion and one minute later is less than about 15 beats per minute, *you have a seriously compromised heart that is biologically older than you are!* Your efforts to improve your heart health may be the most important thing you ever do.

Heart rate recovery of less than 15 beats per minute means your heart is older than your chronological age, and is associated with a marked increase in the risk of death.

If the difference is between 15 and 25 beats per minute, your heart's biological age is about the same as your chronological age.

If the difference is between 26 and 35 beats per minute, your biological age is a little younger than your chronological age.

Above a recovery rate of 35 beats per minute, your biological age is significantly less than your chronological age and you're doing something right. Keep doing it.

If you discover that your heart rate drops only by 12 beats or less in one minute, or if you find that trying to reach your target heart rate makes you uncomfortable or feels entirely unfamiliar, you have a heart that is at high risk of heart attack or stroke. In fact, if your heart rate recovery is this poor, you probably already have heart disease to some degree, even if you don't yet have a specific diagnosis. If so, you should take heart repair very seriously. Start by trying to get your body accustomed to activity according to the recommendations below for those who are new to exercise. But you should also make an appointment with a doctor or personal trainer who can help you safely work up a personalized exercise plan.

If you don't even wear a watch, let alone a heart rate monitor, it's important to learn what your heart rate feels like at various levels of exertion so you can exercise at 60 percent or 80 percent of your heart rate maximum for optimal repair. Once you're familiar with your own heart rate, you can use it to tailor your own fitness plan. For example, to lose fat, aim for 60 percent of your maximum heart rate and exercise for a longer period—brisk walking for two hours burns fat more effectively than a short sprint, even at maximum heart rate.

The following guidance is broken down into four groups of recommendations. The first is for people who have never taken their exercise medicine but who need to start exercising as if their lives depend on it (for they certainly do). Next is guidance for those who can maintain heart health with moderate exercise, then recommendations for people who exercise regularly. The last is for people who already have a high level of aerobic fitness but could tailor their exercise for longevity. Find the group that works for you—and get moving!

#1: New to Exercise

You may not have reached 80 percent of your maximum heart rate in many years and would exert yourself this much only if something with sharp teeth were chasing you. If this is you, you probably have a poor heart rate recovery of 15 beats per minute or less.

One of the best ways for newcomers to discover the pleasures of regular exercise while maintaining a safe level of exertion is to join an exercise group or program led by a professional. Such programs have the added benefit of bolstering the important social support aspect of heart health. The problem with trying to improve aerobic health on your own if you're not already familiar with exercise is that a setback could cause more harm than good and an injury could sideline your quest for heart health. Hire a professional to help you through the first months of tuning up your heart—you won't regret it.

In my clinic I see many people who have avoided aerobic activity for most of their lives. Even talking about exercise is uncomfortable for them, but after taking a close look at their imbalances and quickly realizing that exercise is a big part of the solution to their problems, they usually decide to reap the benefits of exercise, and then learn to enjoy it.

Those new to exercise often ask me, "How fast should I run?" or "How far should I jog?" "Moderation. Moderation. Moderation," I usually answer. "Take a walk around the block after dinner, preferably with someone you love, whether it's your spouse or your dog. Just start with a walk. Every day."

A good rule of thumb is to walk at a pace that makes it challenging to carry on conversation with your exercise partner without becoming breathless, but at which you can still talk. This level of output is where you'll find your aerobic threshold and where your target heart rate for optimal heart repair and maintenance is found.

You can progress faster if it feels good to you, but don't feel like you need to. If you don't already have an aerobic exercise you enjoy doing, exercise equipment is probably the best way to start. But eventually you'll want to branch out and experiment with outdoor or social exercise that adds additional healing (and a lot of fun) to your daily exercise dose.

#2: The Moderate Exerciser

You're a moderate exerciser if you're familiar with exercise but only get around to a bit of low-intensity exercise, like walking at a relaxed pace, a couple of times each week. You know this is you if:

- You can endure a high heart rate (80 percent of maximum) only for fifteen minutes or less.

- You can sustain exertion only if your heart rate stays very low.

- You have a heart rate recovery of 15 to 25 beats per minute.

The great thing about starting from this fitness level is that the fruits of your labors will be obvious, dramatic, life-changing, and inspiring in a relatively short time. In many ways, this is the optimal fitness level for feeling the biggest psychological and physical boost from exercise with the least effort. This is also the fitness level of most readers of health books, so chances are good that you fall into this category. It takes a bit more work for women who are new to exercise to get to the point of enjoying exercise, and those who are already aerobically fit may not experience the same rapid boost that you will as you enjoy the benefits of regular aerobic exercise for the first time. When you start feeling lighter, stronger, sexier, and more energetic in as little as ten days, you'll be that much more inspired to continue with your program. It's an incredible feeling to sense your heart growing younger within your body!

Moderate exercisers are good candidates for a self-designed fitness program, but they're still at risk for injury or burnout. The key to a self-designed plan is patience, persistence, and starting slow. Pick a cardiovascular activity that you enjoy—such as cycling, running, treadmill, stationary bike, cross-country skiing, swimming, or hiking—and do it at least four days a week. Six days is even better. Since you need to exercise year-round, if you prefer to exercise outdoors you'll need to develop your skills and diversify your workout. Also remember that an activity that can be done at a very mellow pace needs to be pushed a little—walking slowly just doesn't tune up your vascular system, but a brisk walk is excellent. Ideally, prepare to suffer a little. Get red in the face. Pant. Sweat. For exercise to have a significant protective benefit for your heart and help you turn off those epigenetic SNPs of disease, you want to be able to handle thirty minutes of 60 to 80 percent maximum heart rate, and it's even better if you can sustain that level of exertion for forty-five minutes to an hour.

#3: Healthy Fit

You're healthy fit if you have a heart rate recovery of 25-40 beats per minute, which means you have probably treated your heart pretty well so far. Well done! However, if you have other concerns, including hormonal imbalance, a family history of brain or heart disease, or mood issues, optimizing your exercise to not only sustain heart function but also optimize healing in virtually every system in your body, you would benefit from a healing-focused exercise plan.

To do this, exercise for 45 minutes at 60 to 80 percent of your aerobic maximum, six days per week. Yes, that means pretty much every day. Consider adding High Impact Interval Training (HIIT), which consists of adding short bursts of high-intensity exercise to your program two to three times per week. Studies have shown that two minutes of HIIT can increase metabolism over 24 hours as much as half an hour of running. Consult with a physical trainer before starting your HIIT program—high impact training has the potential to be, well, high impact in the wrong ways.

#4: The Aerobic Machine

Not many of us fall into this category, but there are particular considerations for the vascular health of those who do. People at this fitness level may have an astounding heart rate recovery of more than 40 beats in one minute. If this is you, your heart health is most likely quite good, provided you also eat a diet low in inflammatory foods and high in fruits, vegetables, fish, and/or grass-fed beef.

You may be an incredible aerobic athlete, but even elite athletes need to pay attention to their long-term heart health. One issue is longevity. Many athletes enjoy incredible fitness during the peak of their careers, but once the buzz of performance and competition wears off, if they hit the sofa and rest on the laurels of their former greatness, they gain weight, lose fitness, and increase their heart disease risk.

A second issue is premature wear on the heart—studies have shown that extreme aerobic athletes have stiffer (older) arteries than people who exercise regularly but not obsessively. Just Google the professional marathon runner Jim Fixx, who dropped dead from a heart attack. His is not an isolated case. Extreme cardiovascular output is hard on the heart.

A third issue for aerobic athletes is that their caloric expenditure can disguise poor nutrition. A less active person eating the same foods would grow overweight and have other warning signs, but an athlete can appear lean and fit while still having high triglycerides, dangerous cholesterol levels, angry hot visceral fat surrounding their organs, and insulin sensitivity.

If you're an aerobic machine, don't stop pursuing your athletic goals, but do remember that you'll need to save some enthusiasm (and cartilage) for maintaining vascular health once your competitive career is over. The good news is that you are well on your way to preventing heart disease—provided you pace yourself to keep up the aerobic exercise for, oh, the next half a century.

Law #3: Get Adequate Sleep

Now that we've covered nutrition and exercise, arguably the two most important parts of heart health, the Precision, Personalized Solution can pick up the pace. The next of Galen's laws is about adequate sleep. This law seems straightforward and obvious—we all want high-quality and adequate sleep. But here is how sleep is uniquely important for heart health, as well as some tips for making sure you catch those ZZZs.

Sleep and Heart Health

Dreams are a sign of rapid eye movement (REM), or deep sleep, which we all need for physical and mental restoration. The REM cycle is crucial for health. Studies done in the 1950s that deprived college students of REM sleep for a week (and were somehow approved) found—surprise, surprise—that they all became severely depressed! During the average night, our bodies go through four to six sleep cycles, and REM sleep is the last part of each cycle. The first REM period is only a few minutes long, but with each cycle the REM duration increases. The dream you wake up remembering is from this last REM cycle. This is the recovery sleep, for all aspects of your body, including your heart.

It's okay if you don't remember your dreams specifically, but if you don't have any sense of dreaming at all, you may not be getting adequate, restorative REM sleep. If you feel that sleep quality is one of your core problems, consider using a wearable sleep quality tracking device.

Why Women Aren't Sleeping

There are two primary reasons why so many women find it difficult to get a good night's sleep, the adrenal hour and sleep apnea:

The "adrenal hour"

Many authors have identified the international sleep crisis in our world, but few have noted the disproportionate suffering of women. In my practice, women are far and away more likely to be getting up with a baby, pacing, or sacrificing their sleep for the sake of a partner or a family member. The special harmony needed in a woman's hormonal symphony also makes her more vulnerable to adrenal dysregulation due to poor sleep. The "adrenal hour," as it's known in Chinese medicine, is a common cause of women waking up at 2:00 or 3:00 a.m.—and being not just awake but wide awake. Their wakefulness is part of the fight-or-flight evolutionary response to protect themselves and their children during prehistoric days—that may seem overreactive in the modern world. Today it's not saber-toothed tigers but modern-day stress that roars at night. A cortisol drop initiates a blood sugar plummet that causes an adrenaline surge to bring sugar to your brain, which wakes you up, for an hour or more, sabotaging not only your night but making you tired the next day as well. This vicious cycle can lead to burnout and mood disorders.

Sleep apnea

Like heart disease, sleep apnea is ignored in women's health—but it's their single biggest heart attack death risk! Sleep apnea occurs when you stop breathing momentarily, or you breathe very shallowly during sleep, resulting in inadequate oxygen delivery. Ask your bedmate, if you have one, to watch for this pattern.

I was taught in medical school that sleep apnea is mainly a concern for men (sound familiar?) who are short and obese and have a thick, short neck and a tongue large enough to block the airway. Obese and overweight people do have an increased risk for sleep apnea, but even the "skinny fat" women we identified earlier can have it too. For both women and men, sleep apnea is a far stronger predictor of sudden death from heart attack than any cholesterol test marker. I test nearly all my patients, especially those experiencing fatigue or stubborn inability to lose weight, with an inexpensive home oxygen device that easily identifies sleep apnea and low oxygen at night.

Sleep apnea sabotages the beautiful harmony of the health symphony, throws hormones out of balance, increases inflammation in the gut, reduces daytime energy, and causes body fat to "hibernate" and become resistant to all weight loss efforts. If you feel that sleep apnea is a core problem for you, your Precision, Personalized Solution needs to include losing weight, eliminating alcohol and smoking, and getting daily exercise.

Tips for Getting Optimal Sleep

The Dr. Mark Sleep Ritual, which I put together after gleaning information from several patients' expensive visits with sleep specialists is a fifteen- to twenty-minute ritual prior to bedtime that includes several steps that will teach your body and brain to sleep soundly all night.

- The first lesson is to sleep only in bed, not in a comfy chair or on the couch. If you want to use a natural sleep support supplement, take it before you start the ritual. Melatonin and tryptophan are natural sleep aids that work for many people, but the quality and dose of these aids are key (see Chapter 8).

- Avoid caffeine and sugary drinks before bedtime (as much as twelve hours before for some people), and don't drink alcohol in the last hour before bed.

- Twenty minutes before going to bed, drink a small amount of chamomile or relaxing decaf tea. (Don't drink too much or you'll be up all night going to the bathroom.)

- Take a warm shower or bath with calming (and non-toxic) essential oils. Lavender is the best. If you don't have time, put a warm washcloth on your face with a little essential oil on it. Then sit back, breathe deeply, and relax.

- Sit in a chair and read a book or magazine, but avoid television, Kindle, your phone, and other screens (blue light from screens is detrimental, particularly to sleep). The thirty medical journals I read each month are better than any sleeping medicine.

- Curl up in a cozy, comfortable bed—again, with no electronics (yes, that means no TV or Netflix on your tablet)—do a few sets of five belly breaths (see "Breathing for Healing" on page 252), and fall asleep.

- If you can't fall asleep, or if you find yourself wide awake later in the night, get up and go back to the chair, read until you feel tired, and then go back to bed.

Some sleep experts recommend that you allow no electronics of any kind in the bedroom in order to achieve optimal sleep. I have found this advice to be helpful for myself, and I tell my patients that the bedroom should be a sacred space for sleep or sex only. Don't have a bedroom TV, don't eat in bed, and keep your smartphone in another room or away from the bed.

Law #4: Drink the Right Fluids

This should be simple: just drink clean water. But even this simple task is becoming harder due to the toxins in our environment, alcohol to relieve stress, and the vitamin and energy drinks promoted by high-profile athletes that are nothing but sugar water. Also don't underestimate the sabotaging power of caffeine in coffee, certain teas, and soda.

I recommend half an ounce of water per pound of body weight per day. If you weigh 150 pounds, then you need 75 ounces of water. That is the equivalent of a six-pack of water (not beer).

Not everyone needs the same amount of water to stay hydrated, but you'll know when you get it right because you'll feel good. The simplest way to get rid of most headaches is to drink water. Try one week of filling your tank with water and see how you feel—probably better than you could with any medication or supplement.

Another aspect of hydration is that each caffeine or alcoholic drink counts as minus two: for each glass of wine or cup of coffee you drink, you lose the equivalent of two glasses of water, owing to the diuretic effect of these drinks, which sneakily pull water out of your body. Ever had a hangover from a night of imbibing and dancing? The toxin of alcohol is part of it, but the dehydration caused by being active without hydrating also contributes to the hangover.

One of my female patients came in with her trusty water bottle (ten years ago before it was trendy) and taught me how she makes sure to drink half an ounce of water per pound of body weight. She bought a 32-ounce water bottle and, since she weighed 160 pounds, filled it up two and a half times a day to get 80 ounces. She reminded me of the importance of BPA-free plastic and said she used a stainless-steel water bottle first, then moved to an all-glass one with a soft neoprene cover.

She also had a $5,000 alkaline water attachment on her kitchen sink that made her drinking water more alkaline and therefore, theoretically, healthier. Squeezing a lemon in your water works just as well, but many women who have these systems praise them. This client also had a reverse osmosis water system in her home that cost $10,000, but she had not had her water tested beforehand. Again, this seems like a large investment with unclear return. Nevertheless, getting your water tested is becoming ever more important. When I had my water tested when I lived in Arizona, I discovered that the lead level was high from the old piping in the house, as was the arsenic level, which supposedly came from the croplands next to us.

This launched my investigation into all sorts of water systems. My conclusion was that the plastic bottled water you buy at the store may not be your best choice, as it may have sat on a pallet in the sun at a warehouse, where the warmth could have caused BPA from the bottle to leach into the spring water and create a bottle of hormone-disrupting water instead of spring water. In addition, recent studies have shown that many bottled water supplies are simply tap water.

At the very least, install a filter on your tap, and if you go the reverse osmosis route, which is the cleanest option, be sure you are replacing the minerals you are removing with organic foods and/or a mineral supplement.

Law #5: Daily Bowel Movement (and Daily Fast)

Earlier I mentioned that the different disciplines of medicine around the world and from different cultures, times, and languages seem to share many of the same health mantras, or messages. One of their most consistent messages is the importance of regular daily bowel movements.

Ayurvedic medicine from India recommends having a morning bowel movement to dispel the toxins from the day before, and this is how I explain it to my patients. So many factors contribute to healthy bowel movements. Yes, it's about the food you eat and how much water you drink, but we also must consider factors related to the history and emotionality around bowel function.

First and foremost is to eat enough fiber. All of us need the right amount of fiber, and over-the-counter drugstore wafers are not the best source. Many of the women I see use fiber wafers for constipation issues and were recommended the wafers by their doctors.

Most women who come to see me are shocked to learn that abnormal gut health and constipation issues are not normal or healthy—and that they're fixable! So many women deal with this, and the Precision, Personalized Solution—fix the gut, fix the heart—has helped thousands of them. Recently, a US government report suggested that over 50 percent of Americans are deficient in magnesium, which supports over three hundred processes in the body—especially in the bowels. And guess what's my favorite nutrient for the heart? Yes—magnesium!

In my clinic we use a special triple blend of magnesium that you take at night (**www.menoclinic.com/supplements**). The triple magnesium blend has magnesium oxide, citrate, and malate—a combo that seems to have a calming effect on mood, helps deepen sleep, and allows for a morning bowel movement to clear toxins. We start with one to two pills at bedtime; if that dose doesn't work, we may go to three for a while; if bowels become too loose, we taper back to one to two pills at bedtime for the optimal once-a-day bowel movement. Of course, you still need your fiber, but get it from organic vegetables, not the drugstore wafer.

I am a fan of fasting, and cleanses, but only if done the right way. We talked about intermittent fasting earlier: finish eating by 6:00 p.m. and fast until fifteen hours later and have breakfast at 9:00 a.m. Emerging research suggests that if you can extend your fast to 16 or 18 hours, you will benefit from increased immune system strength, decreased inflammation, improved hormone balance, and optimized metabolism. Some women do really well on a twenty-four-hour cleanse or fast. But be careful! In my opinion, many of the gimmicks, shortcuts, cleanses, and fasts out there are too aggressive. Too often they simply trick the body for a short time, and then you fall right back into your usual pattern.

Another potential problem is the use of laxatives, which are over-used in our culture. Sometimes we have to "wake up" the bowel after chronic laxative use, and this may take some time. The keys to digestive health and regularity are proper mineral balance (especially magnesium), optimal hydration, and healthy fiber sources from food. Have patience. These recommendations will soon put you on the right path.

Law #6: Control Your Emotions

By now you're well aware that stress is a major insult to your heart health, and Galen's suggestion that we control our emotions is rooted in the stress response. We know that everyone's solution will be different. Some people find great stress relief in a night of dancing, while for others it would be the most stressful night of the year. Assess and change your lifestyle to reduce your own stress, in your own way. Some methods that have worked for my patients include:

Developing an imagery routine (imagine life, better)

Journaling

Meditating

Learning a new sport (especially Zen sports like martial arts, climbing, archery, and yoga)

Finding a different job

Finding a different partner

Developing new friendships

Stress management isn't easy, and it can require making dramatic and sometimes painful decisions. But if you can't reduce your stress to a manageable level, it will kill you. Isn't your life worth making those changes?

Breathing for Healing

Since deep breathing practice seems to help everyone manage stress, I teach my patients how to do "breathing for healing." Sure, we all know how to breathe, but breathing for healing is different. Have you meditated before? Most people never have, but if you have, you already know about breathing for healing. My version is just easier to integrate into your daily life and works well for road rage, work or family challenges, or any other source of stress that makes you anxious. It also helps you resist cravings, such as for junk food or cigarettes. Try it—it works!

Sit back, put your hand on your belly button, and take a deep breath. Did your shoulders go up and the hand on your belly button not move very much? That means it was not a healthy breath, as you used very little of your lungs.

Now take a deep breath while trying to push your hand out with your belly and relax your shoulders. Usually it takes four or five tries before you can take a deep breath keeping your shoulders down and making the hand on your belly move.

Next, breathe in, to a count of five and breathe out to a count of five. Do this three times. Breathe in through your nose and out through your mouth, with your tongue pressed against the roof of your mouth so the air whooshes around your tongue.

Guess what? You just meditated!

Before each meal, sit at the table, say a prayer if that fits your belief system, and take three deep, five-second, in-and-out belly breaths. This will help not only your mental state but also, in very physical ways, prepare your body for food. Breathing for healing primes the digestive system for optimal food digestion by both relaxing and stimulating the organs involved in eating. Three simple five-second belly breaths will do wonders to help optimize your digestive system and release stress—stress that by now you well know is not "just in your head."

Law #7: Breathe Fresh Air

One of my own most powerful medicines is living in Jackson Hole, Wyoming. When I step off a plane after lecturing to doctors in a large city, sleeping in a hotel room, breathing city air, and sitting in airplanes and airports, the amazingly clean, fresh, and vibrant air of my home rushes in to greet me. I can literally taste the difference, and with several deep breaths, I am instantly revitalized. Every morning, I go out on the deck to meditate and I let that cool, clean mountain air talk to every cell in my body. This may seem a little weird, but it is real.

I try to take some time off on the Monday after a lecture weekend to reconnect to the environment and reaffirm why I work so hard to raise my kids in this beautiful place. I feel the same way when I go back home to my birthplace in Nebraska and run in the hills by the river where I used to train for soccer as a kid. I try to connect to the

254 Heart Solution for Women

joy and good energy of that place, and driving down the street to my mom's house, where I grew up, reconnects me with being a kid there. I *consciously* let all the good memories of those times bring me joy.

My favorite bad-air story is the one I tell my kids about living in Phoenix during my medical training. I loved my time there, the people I worked with were amazing, and the care was outstanding. The air quality, not so much. You could see the dirt and smog cloud hanging over the city every evening. Since we could only afford to live in the center of the city, we were smack dab in the middle of the haze. We grew a garden, and when it was time to harvest the cauliflower, the normally bright white heads were orange-brown from the smog. So I cut one off, went to Whole Foods at 5:00 a.m. to buy a beautiful, white, organic cauliflower, and hot-glued it to the plant stalk so I could wake up the kids to "harvest" our cauliflower. They still love this story, but now they know why the cauliflower heads weren't white—until harvest day.

My mantra is clean air, clean food, and clean water, and my first recommendation is to do everything you can to support them. Some things we can't change—like living in Phoenix for medical training—but others we can. We can choose to consume the cleanest food and water possible, install a home air filter, minimize the chemicals we put in and on ourselves, and if we get the chance, we can move to a place with a healthier environment.

Galen's Seven Laws: A Healing Primer

I hope by now you have decided on several areas of your health where you'll focus your healing efforts to reduce your heart disease risk and improve your life. The first time I meet a new patient, I like to give her recommendations for how she can begin solving her problems that very day, and I hope this modern exploration of Galen's seven laws has done the same for you.

The science behind functional medicine therapies are complex, but the implementation is often grounded in common sense and easy to apply to daily life with little more than your intimate understanding of your own body and awareness of the fundamentals of functional medicine that we've talked about so far. The next part of the Precision, Personalized Solution, however, is best undertaken with a critical eye for misinformation and an awareness of your body's unique response to biochemical influences. It's time to learn how to use nutritional supplements. The potential healing value of using nutritional supplements properly is incredible, but reaping the rewards requires figuring out what's right for you. That's why I've dedicated an entire chapter to helping you understand them—focusing, of course, on the ones that are most useful for healing and protecting the heart.

Chapter 8

Targeted Supplements

I prescribe supplements every day, but my ultimate goal is always to use them in ways similar to how I prescribe drugs: as a transitional tool to get my patients to the point where they can maintain health without them. Most of my patients are able to reduce their use of supplements after a certain period, or even eliminate them altogether. Also, so you know where I'm coming from on this, I am not one of those practitioners who's a big fan of supplements and opposed to drugs. To me, drugs and supplements are the same thing—medicine. If we replace a drug with five supplements that don't have the desired results, we are not really succeeding. The goal in my practice is to get my patients to the point where they don't need either drugs or supplements. The key is to think of a supplement as just that: not as an *alternative* to good nutrition and a healthier lifestyle—same goes for drugs. As Hippocrates famously said, "Let food be thy medicine and medicine be thy food." I like to add, "And let your kitchen be your pharmacy and lifestyle your physician."

In a perfect world, making food choices that prevent cellular inflammation and lifestyle choices that strengthen the heart would be enough to prevent heart disease, and for many of us, this is in fact enough. However, we don't get to choose our genetic history, the environment we were born into, or the food and exercise cultures of our childhoods. In addition to these aspects of our lives that are out of our control, our work and living situations often subject us to systemic stress and poor nutrition that can seem nearly impossible to escape. These less-than-ideal conditions can require new weapons in the fight for vascular health: drugs and supplements.

When you are thinking about using supplements, look first for their naturally occurring forms in food as much as possible. Prepare your own food from fresh ingredients (one of the best disease prevention strategies of all time) and add curries, fresh garlic, cinnamon, and ginger to your weekly menu. You can also use these therapeutic foods strategically, increasing their consumption, for instance, after the holidays, after eating a bit of junk food on a road trip, or anytime you feel your body needs a healthy dose of anti-inflammatory goodness.

If you are at low risk for vascular disease, generous consumption of the food sources of these supplements, in combination with a low-inflammation and heart health–conscious lifestyle with plenty of exercise, should be enough to prevent heart disease. If you're like most of us, however, you do have some risk factors for heart disease and will benefit from some well-considered use of nutritional supplements in their concentrated, nutraceutical form.

Supplement Quality

Supplements and herbs are not regulated with the same exacting standards as pharmaceuticals, and their quality varies widely. In 2015, the New York attorney general demanded the removal of supplements from four big-box stores where four out of five of the supplements sold, according to tests, contained *none* of the supplements listed on their labels. You read that right: they contained zero amounts of the active ingredients claimed! We've known for a long time that there is a wide range of quality in supplements, but this was a new low. The pills were stuffed with cheap fillers, including powdered rice, houseplants, and even ingredients, such as peanut powder, that could be dangerous for people with allergies. One of the supplements that claimed to be ginkgo biloba to help memory was actually radish powder.

I hate to have to say this, because I'm a huge fan of natural medicines, but it's the Wild, Wild West in the world of supplements and herbs. Companies are allowed to sell just about anything they can put in a capsule or tablet and to say whatever they want about it. Even when the supplement contains the appropriate ingredients, those ingredients may have been sourced from outdoor labs in India or China where money may not have been spent on quality control and raw ingredients may not have been monitored for heavy metals and toxins.

Aside from the quality of the active ingredients, some of the most popular supplements are so full of binding agents that the tablets go completely through your intestines without breaking down. One of the most popular multivitamins on the market (I won't name names, but it claims to be the number-one vitamin recommended by doctors) has a reputation for coming out the bottom end looking exactly like it did when it went in.

I learned about this when my first day working in the intensive care unit in the St. John's Medical Center in Jackson Hole, one of the ICU nurses approached me and asked if I was the "new nutrition doctor." She then held out a bedpan and as she shook it I could hear the something rattling in the pan. "What's that?" I asked.

"Oh, that's the common vitamin prescribed by doctors, so patients bring them in with them and we call them 'bedpan bullets,'" she replied.

Later, talking to a plumber who came to see me as a patient, the topic of supplement quality came up. I told him the story of bedpan bullets and about some supplements being so tough as to be nearly impossible to digest. "Oh, I know those," he replied. "We find them all the time when we're cleaning out clogged toilets and clearing septic tanks." I have even seen X-rays of patients' intestines showing the undigested vitamins—sometimes with up to six tablets undigested in the small intestine alone.

Packed as some supplements are with binders, preservatives, fillers, and flavor enhancers, your digestive system, depending on how robust it is, may not even break down the pill at all. When you look at your bottle of supplements, you want to see just a couple of ingredients. For example, there are forty-six "other ingredients" listed on the label of that common multivitamin featured in the bedpan bullet story.

Not long after I started my clinic, but before we developed our own supplement line, one of my patients brought in a smoothie she claimed had been purchased from my clinic supply. It had a two-year-old expiration date from a company I trusted. At first, we wondered if we had sold her a two-year-old product, but that wasn't possible. We fill orders monthly, and nothing on our shelves is more than three months old! She swore that she bought it from us, but when we traced the serial number on the bottle, it turned out that she had bought it from an unscrupulous website that sometimes sold expired supplements.

That was the last straw. I decided to start my own line of supplements so that I would be sure to have the highest-quality and freshest supplements on hand for my patients. It was one of the best decisions I ever made for my clinic. We have chosen well-known manufacturers and use only the highest-quality raw ingredients. Before they are manufactured into a final product, these ingredients must pass through up to thirty inspections for quality, purity, and activity.

The very same supplements I prescribe my patients are available online at **www.menoclinic.com/supplements**. Look at our ingredients lists: they usually cite only a few ingredients, the supplement itself and the gelatin capsule. That's it. If you're going to take supplements, this is the kind of quality you want. In fact, one reason why supplements have gotten a reputation for being ineffective is that people take low-quality supplements that don't work.

Some patients come into my clinic with suitcases full of supplements whose ingredients lists they've never even looked at. My first step with a patient who takes a lot of supplements is to have her stop taking all of them for a week. Then we start over, making sure she's taking high-quality supplements that are right for her biochemistry.

My favorite example of how counterproductive it is to skimp on supplement quality is the story of a professional athlete who came into my clinic with poor vascular health indicators across the board. He knew he had issues and was trying to take omega-3 fish oil, but the supplement gave him heartburn and his girlfriend said it gave him bad breath and wouldn't kiss him on the days he took it. I gave him our high-quality fish oil, which uses a triple-distillation process for purity. He called me four days later and said, "My girlfriend says I don't have bad breath anymore, she'll kiss me anytime now, and I can take it without heartburn." Although he was making over $20 million a year, he was saving money by buying his fish oil in large quantities at a grocery store, and it was rancid from day one—already oxidized—and actually bad for his vascular health . . . not to mention his love life.

If you get the good stuff, taking omega-3 supplements is one of the best things you can do for your body. I've seen miraculous things happen with omega-3, but fish oil can also be one of the most toxic items you can buy in a grocery store. Fish oil extracted out of leftover fish parts from Central American fisheries is very different from fish oil extracted from small fish caught in the North Sea or in the cold waters of South America, then processed with special purification manufacturing techniques. Buying good fish oil takes research; the quality of the oil, the toxicity of the contents, and the freshness of the ingredients can be all over the charts.

This extreme variation in supplement quality is enough to make you want to steer away from supplements entirely, but don't despair. The following information will help you tell the difference between the good, the bad, and the ugly as you do your research.

There are three levels of supplements and vitamins:

- Supermarket grade: Includes most multivitamins sold through grocery store chains

- Health food store grade: Includes the common varieties sold at the average health food store

- Nutraceutical grade: Supplements with nutrients derived from food sources, using pharmaceutical-quality control standards

As you consider nutraceutical-grade supplements, visit the website of the Meno Clinic Center for Functional Medicine, open up the web page on supplement quality (**www.menoclinic.com/supplements**), and compare the supplement you are considering with ours.

Some companies analyze supplement ingredients and batches at various points in the manufacturing process and make excellent, pure supplements to which you can trust your life. Buying them, unfortunately, often entails more than just stopping by your nearest health food store or big-box pharmacy.

What Will Supplements Do for You?

The pushers of supplements have created a health problem that is your problem as an individual as well as my problem as a doctor. You don't know what is right for you, and doctors often don't know what their patients are taking. There may seem to be no harm in popping any old vitamin pill every day, but the evidence tells a different story.

Pick up any health magazine in the supermarket and you'll see dozens of advertisements claiming that supplements will do certain things for you, and probably more than a few editorials about supplements that prevent this or do that. All these claims may be right—for some people. But you don't know if they're right for you.

Iron is a great example. Iron is frequently touted as an important mineral for women—and it is. But most iron supplements on the market contain 60 to 300 milligrams of iron and your body needs only 20 milligrams a day. Excess iron makes your body susceptible to bacterial infection, and some scientists have implicated excess iron as a cause of heart disease and cancer. Cooking with a cast-iron skillet may give you all the iron your body requires, but if you took the advice of the supplement companies and health media, you'd be taking an iron supplement every day that contains several hundred times more iron than you need. Even though some supplements are relatively harmless in large doses, I'd go so far as to say this about all supplements: find out if you're deficient before taking them in larger doses than the standard recommended daily allowance (RDA).

Melatonin is another example. The first client I ever prescribed melatonin for had already tried it for insomnia. She'd bought it at the grocery store, and it didn't work. A year of sleepless nights later, she came to me and I gave her some nutraceutical-grade melatonin—it worked like a charm. But just because it worked for her doesn't mean it will work for you. Melatonin works for 50 percent of my patients. It has no noticeable effect on 40 percent of them, and taking it makes 10 percent of them hyperactive and keeps them awake—the exact opposite of the intended result.

Everyone is going to react somewhat differently—and some people dramatically differently—to supplements, drugs, and medical interventions. I wish I could give you a simple cocktail of supplements that would prevent heart disease in everyone, but even with a full workup and all the data from blood tests, we still don't know exactly how people are going to react to a specific supplement until they try it.

I can wholeheartedly recommend that almost everyone take a nutraceutical-grade multivitamin every day—one with the most bioavailable versions of its ingredients—but beyond that, I would caution you to not let the claims of any article, website, or even friend convince you to begin supplements that you have not researched. Always treat supplements the same way you would treat a prescription drug—study the literature on it before taking it, keep a critical eye on your results and side effects to see if it works for you, and then adjust your therapy accordingly.

Unintended Consequences of Taking Supplements

When I was in my internal medicine residency, a gentleman came in for an abdominal aorta repair—a major surgery. During the operation, he began bleeding uncontrollably and eventually went through 112 pints of blood—eleven times his own blood volume. Nobody knew why this happened. I asked his wife about the vitamins and supplements he took. Every day he was taking:

10 garlic tablets

10 vitamin E tablets

10 vitamin A tablets

Over 50 grams of omega-3

This combination synergizes to become a powerful blood thinner, and nobody asked what supplements he was taking or told him to stop these supplements before surgery—which almost killed him.

The unintended consequences of taking supplements could take up an entire book, but here are a few related to heart health:

- St. John's wort is a popular antidepressant among the naturo-pathic crowd—but it causes birth control to become ineffective. And you thought you were depressed before . . .

- Glucosamine, the popular joint health supplement, increases bleeding times by causing warfarin, a blood thinner used in surgery and over the long term to prevent blood clots, to be metabolized more slowly. Don't take glucosamine if you're on blood thinners!

- Chromium picolinate has become a popular weight loss and mood aid, but if you're taking diabetes medication, chromium picolinate may cause your blood sugar to plummet and you'll pass out.

- Calcium supplements should be avoided by some people. If you are not calcium-deficient and you're also taking vitamin D, calcium has no benefit and may put you at greater risk for stroke.

- Poor-quality protein powders, when used by people whose dietary protein intake is already adequate (and most of us do eat plenty of protein), cause undue stress on the kidneys and reduce calcium in the body. The result can be calcium-deficiency disorders and an increased risk of kidney failure in patients with kidney damage.

- Bitter orange, an herbal ingredient in many weight-loss supplements, causes high blood pressure and a racing heart.

- Taking supplements can also lead to what psychologists call the "licensing effect"—the attitude that taking supplements makes it okay to indulge in unhealthy behavior.

- Alpha tocopherol is only one kind of vitamin E, and it's not effective. Some studies have shown that taking alpha tocopherol increases the risk of heart failure, even as other types of tocopherols offer significant vascular protection. Take the right vitamin E—beta, gamma, and delta tocopherols all offer vascular protection. Taking the alpha also blocks the action of the more helpful gamma and delta.

As far as regulation goes, the US Congress has directed the FDA to assume that supplements are safe until proven otherwise. (I'd like to have a word or two with the genius who came up with that one!) Also, supplement manufacturers can put whatever claims they want on their labels, and there is no requirement that they post side effects. They get in trouble if they put in the capsule something entirely different from what the label says, but that's about the extent of supplement regulation. To me, this is the only real difference between drugs and supplements: drugs are subject to considerable oversight from regulatory agencies; supplements are not.

Supplements for Life

I'm a huge fan of supplements and prescribe them daily in my practice—but only after doing an exhaustive study of the patient's deficiencies and designing targeted therapies for her, using the highest-quality supplements combined with lifestyle medicine. If modern medicine were in tune with the proper use of supplements, I'd tell you to just visit your family doctor and do what she or he tells you to do. Unfortunately, however, many doctors have only a rudimentary understanding of supplements, their side effects and complications, and their incredible benefits. That said, a sea change is under way in medicine: many doctors are now bolstering their skills with a more holistic approach to medicine, including the use of supplements.

In my opinion, medicine will eventually evolve to the point where individuals tell their doctors what they need and the doctor's role will be to compare the individual's assessment to the scientific data, deliver recommendations and access to technology, and ensure that the treatment is applied correctly and safely. This paradigm will replace the current one in which, after a 15-minute visit, the doctor is expected to be an all-knowing conveyor of perfect medicine that works the same for everyone (which is impossible).

Until then, let's look at these supplements and learn more about what they will and won't do for your heart health. The following information is presented differently than the information presented in the previous two chapters. There my discussion of some of these supplements was based on their therapeutic potential for an individual's unique body type or core imbalance. The information here is presented in the form of a guide for deciding how to use them and what to consider when you buy them.

Omega-3

Omega-3 fatty acids verge on the miraculous—with an asterisk. They are best consumed with the fish attached; supplemental omega-3 is not as beneficial as eating fatty fish. The supplements also must be fresh and manufactured according to the highest standards. Europe has quality standards for fish oil, but the United States does not (thanks again, Congress). The other well-known source of omega-3, flaxseed oil, contains fatty acids that are much harder for your body to convert to EPA and DHA.

Then there's the troublesome impact on ecosystems. Since omega-3s became popular dietary supplements, overfishing in the oceans has increased. Krill, a small sea plankton creature common in the Southern Ocean, was once viewed as too small to be of interest to fisheries, but they're now harvested by the trillions for their rich omega-3 content. Krill and other fish that were plentiful before the omega-3 health craze, as well as the fish and whales further up the food chain that rely on these omega-3-rich species for food, are now potentially threatened. Some omega-3 oils, however, are derived from fish in sustainable ways, using the parts of fish that are usually discarded after removal of the fillets for food.

If you're going to use fish oil, spend the money on high-quality, sustainably harvested fish oil that is guaranteed not to contain heavy metals and environmental toxins. Even better, eat sustainably harvested, cold-water fish two to three times a week, and if you eat red meat, be sure it's grass-fed beef or game meat, which is also a great source of omega-3. Alaskan salmon, sardines, herring, mackerel, and black cod are excellent sources of omega-3.

Vitamin D

When I worked with Dr. Andrew Weil in Tucson during my internal medicine residency, women would come into the clinic with sun-ravaged faces from sunbathing all day—and yet have shockingly low vitamin D levels below 10. (Vitamin D levels should be over 50 to be considered sufficient.) The problem is that any sunscreen with an SPF (sun protection factor) over 8 blocks all vitamin D absorption from the sun. Now, thanks to our efforts to prevent skin cancer and our indoor lifestyle, most of America is extremely deficient in vitamin D.

Vitamin D is a complex part of our biochemistry. It acts more like a hormone than a vitamin or mineral, and even vitamin D absorbed by the sun is only useful to our bodies after our gut transforms it and our kidneys activate it. Vitamin D is actually a steroid hormone that protects your heart, your brain, and your immune system. You do need the sun to activate vitamin D in the skin, but it's your gut that transforms it into a usable form. Without good gut health, all the sun exposure and vitamin D supplements in the world will not help you.

Vitamin D has been strongly linked to a reduction in heart disease risk, but as we get older, just when we need more of it, our skin loses some of its ability to synthesize vitamin D from the sun. To complicate matters further, we don't find spending time under the sun's harsh rays as pleasant as we did in our youthful days of bronze skin and beach physiques. To utilize the sun's beneficial vitamin D, let the clock be your sunscreen rather than chemicals on your skin. If you must be in the sun for hours, by all means use sunscreen, but a short daily dose of the sun's rays on unprotected skin can be a good thing.

There is no conclusive recommendation on how much sun exposure without sunscreen is safe, and so the best advice is to remember that any coloring is too much. Also, altitude and atmospheric conditions change the intensity of the sun's rays dramatically. Very light-skinned people or people living at higher altitudes may want to limit their daily sun dose to ten minutes or less, and darker-skinned people living at sea level may be safe soaking it up for closer to an hour. A good way to determine what is right for you is to start with ten minutes of exposure. If your skin shows any color at all afterwards, you should shorten your exposure next time. If your skin doesn't show coloring from the sun, you can extend your exposure another ten minutes. Keep adding ten minutes at a time until your find your optimal exposure. Like so many things in our quest for heart health, you have to figure out what is right for you.

Blood tests for vitamin D levels are simple and inexpensive but are not covered by most insurance companies because they don't consider the test "preventative." As usual, insurance companies' definition of what is preventative medicine lags far behind best practices. In my opinion—which is shared by most of my peers—one of the best ways to prevent disease and ill health down the line is to learn your vitamin D level and take steps to optimize it.

Vitamin E

There may be no other supplement that misses the mark more than vitamin E. In one study of 121,000 females between the ages of thirty and fifty-five, supplemental vitamin E (in the form of beta, gamma, and delta tocopherols) was shown to reduce the risk of heart disease by 34 percent. But the alpha tocopherol vitamin E typically available at the supermarket has zero health benefit.

In a revealing demonstration of how woefully out of touch modern medical research is when it comes to vitamins, most studies done on vitamin E use alpha tocopherols. No surprise, then, when these studies conclude that vitamin E shows no benefit.

Vitamin E is essential to a properly functioning body, but vitamin E deficiency is rare. Beta, gamma, and delta tocopherols are powerful antioxidants that help protect our cell membranes from damage and also help our cholesterol do good work rather than harm us. Remember those pesky omega-6 fatty acids? Their inflammatory nature increases your body's vitamin E requirements. Tofu and soybeans, spinach, broccoli, nuts, sunflower seeds, squash, shellfish, and avocado and olive oil are all sources of vitamin E that will do far more for your vascular health than popping grocery store vitamin E pills.

Vitamins B6 and B12 (Methylation)

These are your elite special forces vitamins—the ones you send in to take care of the worst of the undesirables. Of the eight B vitamins, B6 and B12 are proving to be most promising in the prevention of heart disease. These vitamins are being used in nutrient-and-drug cocktails to treat not only heart disease but also homocysteine levels, infertility, mental disorders, osteoporosis, AIDS, bowel issues, skin disease, infection, Lyme disease, and depression, as well as to slow the progression of Alzheimer's. B vitamins convert homocysteine, one of your body's most inflammatory proteins, into methionine, a primary building block for proteins and a healthy part of your system. Without adequate B vitamins, both your homocysteine levels and inflammation increase.

Dietary sources of vitamin B6 include:

- Beans
- Fish
- Poultry
- Dark leafy greens
- Papayas
- Oranges
- Cantaloupe

The kind of B12 you find in most health food store multivitamins is called cyanocobalamin. (The word comes from "cyanide," which should help you remember that this isn't the kind you want.) Cyanocobalamin doesn't exist in nature and is difficult for your body to break down into useful parts, but it's really cheap and easy for pharmaceutical companies to manufacture. For the most part, your body will treat a cyanocobalamin B12 supplement as a waste product and flush it through your system with little to no absorption.

The methylated form of B12 and methyl folate are the compounds we talked about in Chapter 4 that perform the near-miracle of methylation that turns off those inflammatory markers, SNPs, effectively reducing the development of "genetic" disease. You can buy methylcobalamin B12 supplements, but read the ingredient lists to make sure you're getting the methyl version and not the cyano version. Food sources of vitamin B12 are a vegan's worst nightmare: meat, fish, and dairy products. For this reason, most vegans will benefit from a methylcobalamin B12 supplement. Methyl folate is best consumed through cruciferous vegetables like kale, bok choy, radishes, and broccoli. There are methyl folate supplements, but due to potential side effects are best taken under the supervision of a doctor well trained in proper supplement use.

There are many versions of B-complex—B50 and B100, for example—but many are full of binders. Be wary of megadoses of B6, as it can be toxic at high levels; up to 50 milligrams is usually safe. Biotin, included in most high-quality B supplements, can be great for hair and nail growth and quality. Take the gel caps rather than the "horse tablets," which are miserable to take and don't break down very well in the gut. For best absorption, take B12 either alone or as a sublingual (under the tongue).

Methylated B12 is also your most powerful tool for turning off those inflammatory, troublesome SNPs that we talked about earlier. In my practice, I find methyl B12 to be extremely effective at helping people with chronic fatigue, depression, or autoimmune issues achieve a solid base of health and happiness from which they can then work toward heart disease prevention. Methyl B12 is showing promise as a tool for reversing heart disease, and since it's also one of the best tools for preventing inflammation, I'd put good money on it making big news in the very near future as a key part of effective Alzheimer's treatment.

Many processed foods are heavily fortified with folate and B vitamins, but the inflammatory influence of processed and fortified foods outweighs the benefits. A better way to bolster your folate and B vitamin intake than eating fortified but highly processed foods is to take a high-quality multivitamin.

A nutrition plan heavy in vegetables, fish, and grass-fed meat will deliver adequate B vitamins for most people under age fifty. If you're over fifty, you may develop a vitamin B deficiency because reduced stomach acids have made it hard for your body to extract the B vitamins from your food. At this age, the B vitamins in nutraceutical-grade multivitamins are easier for your body to absorb than the B vitamins in food. Although I usually avoid sweeping recommendations on supplements without individual consultation, I will say that just about everyone over fifty will benefit from taking a nutraceutical-grade multivitamin containing methylcobalamin B12 on a daily basis.

Potassium and Magnesium

Potassium is an essential electrolyte that is important for electrical processes in the body, including neural function. It carries a small electrical charge and is crucial to the information exchange in neurons. Every cell in your heart uses potassium to function. Dietary sources of potassium are common, yet low levels of potassium (hypokalemia) are a common electrolyte and fluid imbalance. So if you're getting enough potassium in your diet but suffering from low potassium levels, what's going on?

Nothing in our biochemistry works alone. Excess sodium causes our bodies to excrete potassium, and magnesium allows us to use potassium. This sodium-potassium-magnesium balance is crucial to the nutrient exchange between muscles and the blood, and an imbalance causes significant adverse effects on muscle function, particularly in the heart. In 2010, the USDA reported that over 50 percent of Americans suffer from low levels of magnesium.

If your magnesium is low, your potassium will never recover, and if your potassium is low, your dietary sodium intake will drive up your blood pressure. This is where the confusion about salt intake comes from. "Salt is good," says one expert. "Salt is bad," says another expert. Well, both are right. If your potassium and magnesium levels are healthy, your biochemistry can handle the salt. Unfortunately, most of us consume way too much salt and not nearly enough potassium and magnesium, and that combination drives up our blood pressure, ultimately decreasing the oxygen flow to our hearts.

Kidney and adrenal issues can also limit your body's ability to process potassium, and diuretics, laxatives, and steroids can cause low potassium levels. One of the most common causes of a potassium imbalance is medications, which can cause life-threatening levels, both high and low. The good news is that you won't have to worry about potassium if you take care of your adrenal gland by managing your stress levels and take care of your kidneys by avoiding metabolic issues like diabetes and high blood pressure and eating lots of vegetables and fruits. Most multivitamins contain a small dose of potassium and magnesium.

Medical experts routinely advise athletes and outdoor workers to drink electrolyte replacement sports beverages, which are high in salt and loaded with high-fructose corn syrup. These drinks have two-thirds the sugar of sodas and more than three times as much sodium. In other words, commercial electrolyte replacement drinks may replace some potassium and magnesium but at the same time do more harm than good through the inflammatory effects of HFCS and sodium.

UC Berkeley researchers reported that students who drink one 20-ounce "sports drink" daily for one year will gain about 13 pounds.

I help the athletes I work with by building them an electrolyte replacement drink, Meno Electrolyte, which has the electrolytes in the proper balance of potassium and magnesium with the sodium—and contains no sugar. You can mix your own electrolyte replacement drink using this simple recipe: to each cup of water, add two tablespoons of fresh-squeezed orange juice and one-eighth of a teaspoon of high-potassium salt.

I usually recommend magnesium glycinate for overall health, as it doesn't affect the bowels and works great to reduce the heart palpitations or extra beats many women feel occasionally. Magnesium oxide, which tends to loosen the bowels, is a better option if you tend toward constipation. For optimal sleep, magnesium is best taken at night.

Potassium is a great example of an overused supplement that can cause irregular heartbeats and other serious health problems. If your doctor or anyone else recommends potassium supplements to you, seek a second opinion and also make sure that your potassium levels are monitored during the treatment.

Vitamin K

Vitamin K, mostly found in green vegetables, is so essential to vascular health that, with our increased understanding of biochemistry, the Institute of Medicine's dietary recommendation for this vitamin has been increased by about 50 percent since the 1990s. Retrospective studies have shown that individuals with early-stage Alzheimer's consumed half as much vitamin K as cognitively intact individuals of the same age. Additionally, one of the genetic risk factors for both heart disease and Alzheimer's, the apolipoprotein E4 allele, is associated with lower vitamin K levels. Rats fed a diet low in vitamin K throughout their lives develop cognitive difficulties in old age. In your greater vascular system, vitamin K also helps maintain arterial plasticity, reducing your risk of heart disease.

Vitamin K is not a single vitamin but actually a family of vitamins, K1 to K7, and there are probably many more subtypes in the natural form. Synthetic vitamin K, menadione, can be toxic if taken in high doses, so—surprise, surprise—vitamin K is another vitamin best consumed in food rather than as a supplement. Doing that, however, is the tricky part. Most people, even those with otherwise healthy diets, are deficient in vitamin K, partly because the most concentrated source of it is fermented foods. The Japanese, whose culture is known as one of the healthiest in the world (aside from working so much they have a word for "death by work"), eat a wide variety of fermented foods. In America, unfortunately, fermented foods are limited to items we often view as condiments and don't eat on a regular basis.

To ensure that you are consuming enough vitamin K, don't treat vegetables like garnishes—eat them like a main course. Vitamin K–rich foods include:

- Olive oil

- Soybeans

- Asparagus

- Leeks

- Okra

- Hot spices

- Brassica vegetables (broccoli, cabbage, and cauliflower)

- Green onions

- Herbs

- Fermented foods

We all eat some of these vegetables, but most of us just don't eat enough. Of the K vitamins, we're most likely to be deficient in K1 and K2. K2 is hard to get in the diet. Aged cheeses like brie, gouda, and blue cheese contain K2, and so does foie gras (goose liver) pâté. The food with the most K2 by a large margin is natto, the fermented soybeans popular in Japan. Perhaps vitamin K has something to do with why, France and Japan are second and third—from lowest—on a list of heart disease death rates by country.

For bone density and heart health, metabolism, and functioning, K2 is arguably the most important of the K vitamins, yet it is synthesized in our bodies and not found in substantial amounts in food sources. For this reason, a deficiency in K2 requires supplemental K2. Most of the higher-quality vitamin D supplements now include vitamin K to synergize with the vitamin D for bone health. Vitamin K in some forms can affect the blood thinner coumadin, but the form of vitamin K added to vitamin D supplements seems to carry no risk for people on blood thinners.

Antioxidants

Antioxidants are our primary weapon against the cellular violence of free radicals. If it weren't for the antioxidants produced by our bodies and bolstered with our diet, factors like smoking would kill us a whole lot quicker. Scientists have targeted one antioxidant in particular, glutathione, for protecting the lungs well enough that some smokers can go through a pack a day for many years before it kills them. Glutathione is found in the fluid in the lungs, among other places. Reducing your exposure to free radicals by increasing your antioxidant function needs to be a fundamental basis of your decision-making that will extend the health of your tissues, improve your vitality, and lengthen your life span.

You'll notice that I said you need to increase antioxidant *function* rather than to take antioxidant *supplements*. There is certainly a place for antioxidant supplements, but the data have shown that antioxidant supplements alone do little to decrease the risk of vascular disease, and high doses of certain antioxidants can have negative side effects. Taking a high-quality multivitamin gives you all the supplemental antioxidant you should take without professional supervision. The rest of your oxidative stress reduction should come from the foods you eat and a lifestyle that minimizes free radical exposure.

Antioxidant function is widely misunderstood, and it starts with a grammatical mistake. Most people use antioxidant as a noun, thinking it's something we eat or ingest, and do not understand that first and foremost it's the adjective form denoting the process of antioxidation, as in antioxidant function. Just eating foods or supplements with antioxidant properties does not ensure effective antioxidation in your body. Today's nutritional advice to eat antioxidants to fight free radicals is rudimentary at best.

Functional medicine doctors, using the antioxidation process to develop individualized treatments, have seen results that far exceed the expectations of modern medicine. If you are edging toward disease or already have a disease, taking antioxidants isn't enough. You'll need a custom program designed for you, based on a thorough workup of your systemic deficiencies and excesses, to bolster your body's natural antioxidation capability. To better understand how antioxidants work and choose what's best for you, consider these well-known and lesser-known antioxidant processes:

Melatonin

Melatonin occurs naturally in our bodies. The supplemental synthetic melatonin, which is available over the counter, is best known as a sleep aid, but it is also a powerful antioxidant and anti-inflammatory. In pharmacological doses, under physician supervision, melatonin has dramatic effects. It can lower blood pressure, improve cholesterol balance, restore liver enzymes, and improve insulin function, and it may even bolster mitochondrial function. Melatonin works on a circadian rhythm cycle, helping your body repair and nourish itself during rest. Provided it is not mixed with sedatives, I get excellent results with melatonin, but I do not recommend it for patients with a susceptibility to depression.

Glutathione

My friend and colleague Dr. Mark Hyman has called glutathione "the mother of all antioxidants, the master detoxifier and the maestro of the immune system." In an article in *HuffPost* he explains his reverence for the power of glutathione through his experience as a physician:

> In treating chronically ill patients with Functional Medicine for more than 10 years, I have discovered that glutathione deficiency is found in nearly all very ill patients. These include people with chronic fatigue syndrome, heart disease, cancer, chronic infections, autoimmune disease, diabetes, autism, Alzheimer's disease, Parkinson's disease, arthritis, asthma, kidney problems, liver disease and more.

The protein glutathione is your body's heavyweight antioxidant, and as Hyman notes, genetic deficiency in the gene that triggers glutathione production is a striking commonality in patients with a multitude of diseases, including heart disease. To bolster your glutathione production, eat foods rich in sulfur, the key element in glutathione. Good dietary sources of sulfur include garlic, onion, and cruciferous vegetables like broccoli, collard greens, kale, cabbage, cauliflower, and watercress. And exercise, as you're probably expecting to hear again by now, also boosts glutathione production.

Manufacturing a glutathione supplement is tricky because your body will simply digest the protein. To make the glutathione bioavailable, quality manufacturers use a special fat capsule form called liposome and add supplemental folate and vitamins B6 and B12, which help your body's natural glutathione production. A less expensive way to increase your glutathione level is to take N-acetyl cysteine, a glutathione building block that converts to glutathione in your body.

Exercise as an antioxidant

Perfectly demonstrating that antioxidation is a process rather than a substance is the fact that moderate, frequent exercise is one of our most effective tools in reducing oxidative stress. The increase in free radicals from our muscles' mitochondria triggers our natural antioxidant production. Considering that living things have been engaged in a balancing act with free radicals for billions of years, we've gotten pretty good at it, but our bodies are now subject to new insults that have only been at work since the proliferation of man-made toxins and industrial food processing. Today our antioxidant response has a lot more work to do, but fortunately, exercise remains one of the most beneficial antioxidants available to us.

Dr. Mark's Top Supplement Choices by Body Type

Based on both scientific evidence and my clinical experience, the following supplements have proven effective at helping to heal the imbalances most strongly associated with each of the three body types outlined in the Precision, Personalized Assessment.

The Apple Body Type

Chromium

Chromium has been used for weight loss for decades because it improves metabolism. This trace mineral regulates blood sugar to prevent spikes, and for twenty years it's been my go-to supplement for improving metabolism. Chromium is often combined with vanadium, as there appears to be a synergy of these two minerals in metabolizing sugar.

Dose: 250–500 micrograms per day

Berberine

This is one of my favorite supplements because it has multiple effects and, when combined with chromium, is a game-changer in helping patients with the apple body type avoid medications. Berberine also seems to reduce that dreaded sugar craving.

Dose: 100 milligrams twice per day

Cinnamon

A teaspoon of cinnamon a day keeps the apple body type away. Well, not by itself, but there is evidence that cinnamon can slow down sugar spikes and insulin release. I once had a client do a simple finger-stick blood sugar test for two weeks. The first week she ate her oatmeal without cinnamon, and the second week she ate her oatmeal with cinnamon. Her blood sugar levels were lower during the cinnamon week.

Dose: 200 milligrams per day

Alpha-lipoic acid

Alpha-lipoic acid is an antioxidant that works at the cellular level to reduce insulin spikes by opening the "sugar gates" so that more stored sugar is available for energy use. There are multiple benefits to this antioxidant for the metabolism, blood sugar, the brain, and the nervous system. It has even been shown to reduce diabetic neuropathy, which results from the death of small nerves in the feet due to the blood sugar and insulin spikes.

Dose: 100 milligrams twice per day with meals

Vitamin D3

Almost everyone has low vitamin D levels. Every cell needs it, it increases the efficiency of insulin, and when you need less insulin to process the same amount of sugar, less fat accumulates around the belly. The current guidelines for healthy levels of vitamin D3 in the blood suggest a minimum of 30 nanograms per milliliter (ng/ml), but I prefer to see 60–80 ng/ml in lab results.

Dose: 4,000 IU per day in the winter and 2,000 IU per day in the summer (cut these doses in half if you're very petite or under 110 pounds and consider testing to see if you need such a high dose)

Magnesium

Even the US government stated that over half of America is deficient in magnesium. Why is this deficiency a big problem? Because magnesium is part of over 350 chemical reactions that help the body function more efficiently—just what you need if you tend to store fat around the belly. As I mentioned in the previous section of this chapter, I prefer magnesium glycinate for overall health and magnesium oxide for those with a tendency toward constipation.

Dose: 400–800 milligrams per day, taken at night for improved sleep

Probiotics

Probiotics can reduce your tendency to store fat around the gut, especially the centralized, hot fat of the apple body type. Besides helping you lose body fat, they also optimize communication, improve your efficiency at harvesting nutrition—which translates into fewer transient blood sugar and insulin spikes—and support your gut metabolism. Use probiotics with lactobacillus and bifidobacteria as main ingredients, and don't get tricked by the "billions and billions" sales pitch: quality is more important than quantity.

Dose: One per day

Gymnema and fenugreek

Fenugreek slows down absorption of sugar from the gut and makes insulin work more efficiently. Gymnema has similar effects, and I see real synergy when these two are combined in high-quality supplements. The science supports their use to optimize blood sugar and reduce the damage from insulin. This combination is my go-to supplement to curb carb cravings. It works best as a liquid, although, because of unpleasant taste, most of my patients prefer to use the capsule form.

Dose: 200 milligrams twice per day each

Banaba leaf

This supplement comes from the Southeast Asian banaba tree and contains a special chemical that helps optimize sugar shifts. You will see banaba leaf combined with several of the supplements already described. In my experience, everyone responds differently to such combinations: sometimes these supplements taken together create a synergy where one plus one equals more than two—when you hit the right supplement combination for your biochemistry, sometimes it adds up to ten! This is what I look for in tailoring my recommendations to individuals: those "sweet spots" provided by a synergy of optimal nutrition, exercise, sleep, stress management, and targeted high-quality nutritional supplements.

Dose: 100 milligrams twice per day

The Pear Body Type

Plant-based protein shake/smoothie

The first nutritionist I worked with was a dietitian who had great intentions and training. I did my two-hour interview and exam with the first collaborative care patient we worked on together, and then it was the nutritionist's turn. With all her good intentions and excellent education to back her recommendations, she gave our patient twenty handouts, told her to eliminate casein, whey, gluten, soy, and corn and to drink more water, and gave her fifty recipes for things the patient had never eaten or cooked before.

When I went back in the room thirty minutes later, the woman was crying. Through her tears, she told me that, with her low energy and

The Meno Clinic Smoothie

The Meno Clinic Smoothie (**www.menoclinic.com/smoothies**) is an organic protein smoothie mix that is pea protein–based, not whey- or soy-based. Combine this protein mix with 10 ounces of coconut milk (not coconut water!). Unsweetened coconut milk is best, but you can use the vanilla-sweetened kind if you need sweetener to enjoy it. (The protein in the smoothie will help blunt that dreaded blood sugar spike we so want to avoid.) Finally, add half a cup of frozen organic berries and you have a yummy fruit smoothie for a meal.

I prefer coconut milk over almond milk for several reasons. One, the coconut milk has fatty acids that are good for the skin, eyes, brain, and heart, whereas almond milk, which is essentially almond water, doesn't deliver this extra benefit. And two, after reviewing thousands of food sensitivity test panels, I have rarely seen a coconut sensitivity, yet I see almond sensitivities weekly.

For chocolate lovers, we have a chocolate pea-based protein powder. This one can be mixed with coconut milk, a few pieces of ice, a banana, and a tablespoon of healthy nut butter for a smoothie that rivals any sweet treat at any restaurant.

Use a bullet-type mixer to make a breakfast that takes forty-five seconds to prepare, is yummy, and treats your body to a minimal sugar curve, improved metabolism, no insulin spike, and no inflammation. I have one every day, as do most of my staff, not only because it tastes so good but because, with a nutritious, non-inflammatory start to our day, we feel so good the rest of the day.

brain fog, she could never do what the nutritionist had recommended. Wasn't there an easier way? So I took back all the handouts, told her to close her eyes, and asked her to imagine making a yummy chocolate milkshake for breakfast every day for a month and avoiding bread. Could she do that? She started laughing, thinking I was joking, but I was not. This has been my approach to nutrition for twenty years: start low, have fun, go slow. You can't do it all at once, and you want to find success quickly.

She left that day ecstatic with a thirty-day hormone balance prescription that consisted of:

- An organic, plant-based protein smoothie for breakfast and lunch each day (see the sidebar on the Meno Clinic Smoothie)

- A basic dinner with high-quality, hormone-free protein, a healthy vegetable, and a piece of fruit for dessert

- A probiotic and two supplements

Diindolemethane

One of my favorite supplements for hormonal support, DIM, is essentially "broccoli in a bottle." Cruciferous vegetables like broccoli, Brussels sprouts, cauliflower, and kale contain chemicals that help the body eliminate xenoestrogens, those estrogen-mimicking compounds from the environment that confuse our own hormonal messaging. If you have a pear body type, you should be eating these foods, but consider adding this supplement as well. I also recommend DIM for any of my patients taking supplemental hormones.

Dose: 100 milligrams per day

Vitamin D3

One benefit of vitamin D3, the supplement I prescribe most often, is that it protects the endocrine system against the communication disruptors that cause so much trouble for the pear body type.

Dose: 4,000 IU per day in the winter and 2,000 IU per day in the summer (cut these doses in half if you're very petite or under 110 pounds and consider testing to see if you need such a high dose)

Probiotics

I can't say enough about how these superheroes of the gut help restore balance to the microbiome and hormonal messaging. Eat the prebiotic foods, such as artichokes, dandelion greens, onions, leeks, and asparagus, that feed the probiotics. Use probiotics with lactobacillus and bifidobacteria as main ingredients.

Dose: one per day

Curcumin

Derived from a main phytochemical in turmeric, curcumin reduces inflammation in the body at the cellular level and can help balance estrogen levels. To get enough curcumin from eating turmeric you would have to eat several pounds of it! The pepper derivative piperine is usually added to high-quality curcumin-based products to aid absorption, so look for this on the label. Of all the supplements detailed in this book, curcumin may be the most important. Funny how a nutrient used to promote health for over three thousand years is now being "discovered"!

Dose: 500 milligrams per day, depending on the concentration of curcuminoids, the active ingredient in curcumin

Magnesium

One of the main benefits of magnesium for the pear-shaped body is that it helps you relax, sleep better, and have more regular digestion. Magnesium also regulates cortisol, assists the hormone manufacturing system, and supports energy systems. Use magnesium oxide if you tend toward constipation; magnesium glycinate is best for everyone else. To increase magnesium absorption, many women opt for Epsom salt (magnesium) baths, which I recommend combining with lavender for a more relaxing experience. Go ahead, pamper yourself with a long, warm, soothing lavender Epsom salt bath. You deserve it, and your hormones will thank you for it!

Dose: 400–800 milligrams per day

Licorice root extract

Licorice root extract supports the stress reduction aspect of hormone balance by bolstering cortisol levels. Look for deglycyrrhizinated licorice (DGL), as a component that can elevate blood pressure has been removed from this form of the supplement. (If you are on blood pressure medicine, the DGL version is a must.) DGL is also easily obtained from licorice root tea. It does tend to keep you awake, so drink it before 3:00 p.m. Several of my patients prefer this tea as a morning drink instead of coffee.

Dose: 250–500 milligrams per day, and never more than 1,000 milligrams per day

American ginseng and Siberian ginseng

The herbs American ginseng (*Panax quinquefolius*) and Siberian ginseng (*Eleutherococcus senticosus*) help modulate cortisol levels and can support hormone balance by providing both stimulatory and adaptive benefits to protect from stress. They work by increasing your metabolic rate, which burns the type of fat found in the pear-shaped body. Be aware that some women find them overstimulating.

Dose: 100 milligrams per day, in the morning (read labels carefully because dose and quality vary widely and are brand- and source-specific)

Vitamin B-complex

All B vitamins are critical for proper function of the adrenals and provide multiple other benefits. This is why some B-complex supplements are marketed as "stress support."

Dose: Variable! Usually a blend of B1, B2, B3, B6, B12, and folate at variable doses

L-theanine

L-theanine is a calming amino acid that relaxes the brain and creates a sense of well-being.

Dose: 100 milligrams one to two times per day

Phosphatidylserine

Phosphatidylserine helps to regulate sleep cycles and prevent the dreaded "adrenal hour," a holistic medicine term for the wakefulness many of us experience like clockwork between 1:00 and 3:00 a.m., owing to a sudden cortisol shift.

Dose: 150 milligrams one to two times per day

L-acetylcarnitine

To improve poor circadian rhythm function (better known as "tired and wired but can't sleep") as well as brain and neurotransmitter function, look for a special form of acetylcarnitine called L-acetylcarnitine, which is better at crossing the blood-brain barrier for additional healing.

Dose: 100 milligrams one to two times per day

Ashwaganda and rhodiola

The adaptogenic herbs ashwaganda and rhodiola help to modulate cortisol levels and provide protective armor so that stress does not beat you up further.

Dose: 100 milligrams per day, one to two times per day each

The Skinny Fat Body Type

I do not usually recommend supplements for the skinny fat body type. If this is you, lifestyle factors will help far more than supplements. However, I do strongly recommend that you do two things:

- Get a blood test for vitamin D3 or just start taking the supplement (4,000 IU in the winter and 2,000 IU in the summer, but less if you weigh under 110 pounds) and check your levels by taking a blood test three months later.

- Have your doctor check your bone density starting at age forty-five instead of the standard age of sixty-five. Ask for either a dual-energy X-ray absorptiometry (DEXA) bone scan or, even better, a heel ultrasound version, which is much less expensive and emits no radiation. In this body type, we usually miss a crucial window to reverse bone loss. If your bone density results are abnormal, use natural therapies and food as medicine rather than the medications for treatment. If your bone health is normal at age forty-five, then recheck it every five years.

Dr. Mark's Top Supplements for Heart Support

By this point, you may feel that you have specific heart disease risk but still be unsure about which supplements will heal your imbalances best. If so, consider the following supplement packages. These are the ones I use most and with the greatest success in helping women with elevated heart disease risk. They target heart-specific musculature, gut health, exercise recovery, and the hormones with the closest relationship to heart function. The guidelines here are for my own Meno Clinic brand, which I know will provide optimal quality and results. There are other high-quality varieties out there, but be sure to do your homework to make sure they're as high-quality as the Meno Clinic supplements (**www.menoclinic.com/supplements**).

Coenzyme Q_{10}

High-quality CoQ_{10} uses a micro-emulsion delivery system that allows us to pack high doses of ubiquinone CoQ_{10} in an easy-to-swallow softgel. CoQ_{10} is used to help treat high blood pressure and heart disease, enhances immune system function, and reduces high cholesterol levels in the blood. It also provides an energy boost for people dealing with fatigue.

Carnitine

High-quality carnitine uniquely combines two forms of carnitine, L-carnitine and its acetylated form, into one capsule in an optimal four-to-one ratio. Carnitine plays a critical role in energy production, supports athletic performance, and may speed recovery time from intense exercise.

Ribose Powder

Ribose synthesizes adenine nucleotides, which are required by cardiac muscle and other tissue to make adenosine triphosphate (ATP), the primary source of energy used by all cells to maintain normal health and function. D-ribose supports cardiovascular health and energy levels, especially muscle energy, and improves performance for both athletes and weekend warriors.

Omega-3

High-quality omega-3 supplements (*dose:* 600 milligrams EPA, 400 milligrams DHA) are enhanced with the addition of lipase, a digestive aid, to ensure maximum absorption. Fish oils are harvested from sustainable fisheries, molecularly distilled, and filtered to ensure purity and maximize the removal of heavy metals, pesticides, solvents, and other contaminants.

Vitamin D

Vitamin D3 is essential to bone health, as it promotes intestinal re-absorption of calcium, reduces urinary calcium loss, and supports colon health. Working together, these two benefits maintain healthy serum calcium levels to support bone health, which in turn supports heart health.

Probiotics

High-quality probiotics support the immune system and improve intestinal function. To ensure delivery of the highest number of live organisms to the intestinal tract, the best probiotics are designed for release over an extended time frame (ten to twelve hours), which ensures delivery throughout the entire tract.

Organic Super-Protein

The best protein powders come in natural flavors, provide at least 20 grams of protein per serving, and use natural pea protein isolate, which has more than twelve amino acids and offers high bioavailability and digestibility. The best raw materials for making the protein powder are USDA-certified organic, North American–grown yellow peas, a true vegan protein (gluten-, dairy-, and soy-free) that is not genetically modified (non-GMO) and is produced with a natural fermentation process that uses no chemical solvents.

Glutamine

Glutamine is a major fuel for the intestines and supports the functioning of the gastrointestinal tract. It aids in tissue growth and is the nutrient of choice for maintaining the intestinal mucosal lining.

Glutamine also supports the growth of muscle mass and is known to support the immune system—specifically, the powerful immune system found in the gut.

Digestion Support Supplements

High-quality digestion support supplements blend digestive enzymes with betaine HCL to support optimal digestion of proteins, fats, and carbohydrates. The best brands contain the protease dipeptidyl peptidase IV (DPP IV), which aids in the breakdown of casomorphin (from casein) and gluteomorphin (from gluten), as well as the enzyme lactase, which helps break down the dairy sugar lactose. By reducing the inflammation associated with digestive dysfunction, a digestion support supplement taken before meals may be helpful for those who experience gas and bloating after eating and who tend toward constipation. But before you buy this supplement, try eating a slice of dried mango with your meal. It might work even better than a supplement.

Adrenal Support Supplements

High-quality adrenal support supplements combine whole herbs that nutritionally support the adrenal cortex and glands. By enhancing the body's ability to produce certain adrenal hormones, these supplements support the immune system and also relieve mild stress and frustration.

Thyroid Support Supplements

A high-quality thyroid support supplement is an all-in-one thyroid support product that may benefit many thyroid conditions. Look for non-stimulating, adaptogenic, botanical American ginseng (*Panax quinquefolius*) to help control cortisol variations and serum blood glucose and insulin levels.

If your thyroid is not functioning correctly, nothing else in your body will work efficiently, but thyroid dysfunction is probably the most common, least understood, and most poorly treated issue in all of medicine. Hypothyroidism, the name given to low production of thyroid hormone, is vastly underrecognized. Many of my patients have vague complaints that they attribute to aging, yet healing their thyroid frequently resolves their complaints. We know that for optimal health the thyroid must be balanced so that the rest of the hormonal symphony stays in tune. For example, suboptimal thyroid function worsens insulin resistance, leading to further inefficient blood sugar metabolism and eventually to heart disease (as well as further thyroid dysfunction). There is intimate communication between the thyroid and insulin, as well as between the thyroid, cortisol, and the male and female hormones. Only a personalized approach to breaking the vicious cycle of thyroid dysfunction will be successful. We must look at the entire symphony and understand the interplay to achieve harmony.

One in five women and one in ten men have thyroid problems, yet up to 50 percent of them are undiagnosed, and even those on thyroid therapy are often undertreated. There are two key steps to fixing a sluggish thyroid. The first is getting the right testing to confirm the presence of a thyroid problem. The standard test is the thyroid stimulating hormone (TSH) test, often accompanied by tests of the active form of thyroid hormone (free T3), the inactive form (free T4), and the anti-TPO antibody. The second step is designing a personalized approach to healing your thyroid that provides optimal energy, boosts metabolism, and balances all the other hormones.

Even though there are several different reasons for low thyroid function, many doctors ignore thyroid function and will tell patients experiencing dysfunction, especially women, "You are normal. Just exercise more and eat less and everything will be fine." Or they put their patients on an antidepressant, diabetes medication, or cholesterol medication. In the end, these patients are treated for heart disease—when all along it's the thyroid screaming to be heard.

Thyroid Dysfunction: The Real Culprit

One young woman came to see me with the typical story I hear. Thirty pounds overweight, she could not change her body fat no matter what she did. She ate clean, tried every diet, worked with a personal trainer, and even saw a psychiatrist for her low mood. She wondered if she had fibromyalgia combined with chronic fatigue syndrome and some depression mixed in as well. Her menstrual cycles were irregular, painful, and accompanied by severe mood changes.

The problem all along had been her thyroid. After taking health fair lab tests, she was told that her thyroid was normal, but a more personalized and advanced thyroid evaluation told a different story. Part of the problem for women getting tested for thyroid function is that the endocrine societies have lowered the threshold for what we now diagnose as hypothyroidism, but few labs have adjusted to the new normal.

We designed a personal approach for her that used lifestyle medicine, a proper low-level exercise program, and low-glycemic food based on a personalized nutrition evaluation (testing for food sensitivities showed that dairy was poison for her thyroid) and balanced her adrenals with no need for further testing. And sure enough, she lost weight, her mood improved dramatically, and her pain and fatigue subsided.

If you have a thyroid problem, you will also have an adrenal problem, since they are "sister glands" that talk to each other in ways we are just beginning to understand.

The best way to jump-start your thyroid health is a full body detoxification. In addition to eliminating high-glycemic, processed foods and anything with synthetic hormones and consuming only nutrient-dense simple foods, you can also use a detox package. The one I use in my clinic is the Meno Clinic Plus 14-Day Detox Program (**www.menoclinic .com/cleanse**), but other good ones are out there. I recommend speaking to your doctor about any detox package you plan to use.

Tyrosine

The amino acid tyrosine is a building block for several neurotransmitters, or brain chemicals, that regulate mood, and it's also a building block for the thyroid hormones. Tyrosine is crucial for thyroid health, and for years I simply prescribed tyrosine alone. Now I find that it acts more efficiently when combined with some of the other supplements discussed here. The Meno Clinic Thyroid Support supplement is an easy way to get what you need in the right balance.

Dose: 100–200 milligrams per day

Selenium

Selenium is crucial for converting the inactive form of thyroid hormone (T4) into the active form (T3). Many women are deficient in this nutrient because the soils where our food is grown are very depleted. Even my vegan, healthy, food-conscious, organic food–eating patients seem to come up deficient in selenium and benefit from supplementation. There are times when this supplement alone is the game-changer for thyroid health.

Dose: 50 micrograms per day

Iodine

Iodine is one of the most crucial elements of thyroid function, yet it also gets people in trouble. There seems to be a wide range of opinions on the correct dosing, and a urine test to determine your optimal dosing may be advised. The very high doses prescribed by some doctors make me nervous because, as an internal medicine specialist, I have admitted over a dozen women to the ICU with "thyroid storms."

This happens when a person with suspected thyroid problems takes a large dose of iodine, as recommended, and her thyroid responds by "dumping" all the active hormone and setting off an adrenaline type of effect that leads to the "storm": a racing heart and potentially life-threatening heart rhythm changes. So start low, go slow, and be sure to test your iodine levels before taking large doses of it.

Dose: 20–100 micrograms per day

Chapter 9

Working with Your Doctor to Get Off Pharmaceuticals

The incredible effectiveness of using lifestyle, exercise, food, and supplements as medicines to heal the heart is exciting, but what do we do when nutrition and supplements are no longer enough and we need professional help? And if you've already sought professional help and been prescribed medication that you may or may not benefit from, how do you get off the medication you don't need and start with a clean slate to build your solution?

Well, by now you're probably expecting me to say that every individual is unique. You're right: there is no one-size-fits-all answer to that question. However, there are some guidelines you can use to work with your doctor to fine-tune your solution, use cutting-edge blood tests to reveal your individual imbalances on a molecular scale, get off the drugs you may be taking now, and find the right drugs in the right doses if they're necessary to balance your particular biochemistry.

Before going to see a doctor about your heart health, the first step is to change how you think about medicine. A good example of how to look differently at what your doctor can do for you is the story of Lori, a cattle rancher who came to see me for help with a wide range of problems. But this story isn't about Lori's health—it's about her cows.

Bleeding the Cows

Lori spent her working life running four hundred head of cattle on a ranch in Wyoming. When she came to see me, she was in her mid-fifties and on five medications, including a cholesterol-lowering statin that made her feel weak and depressed after the first week on the drug and a blood pressure medication that, unbeknownst to her, was causing fluid to collect in her feet by the end of the day, which made her feel terrible. She was particularly receptive to my ideas about how she could get off the drugs and replace them with lifestyle therapies and supplements to regain her internal balance. It wasn't until fifteen years later, when we were having lunch together one day, that she told me an incredible story that explained why she'd had no doubt that the personalized approach to balancing her internal system would help her far more than any of the five drugs she was taking.

When she and her husband were running cows on their slice of the Wyoming prairie, they began having serious issues with sickness in their herd, and the ranchers around them were having the same problem. At its peak, Lori recalled, "I had four calves lying on the kitchen floor of our house, each one hooked up to an IV drip, with the IV bags hanging from cabinet doorknobs and drawer handles. The calves were dying from dehydration and malnutrition. After that I told my husband, 'This has to stop.'"

Their local vet was holistically minded and told them that to discover the root cause of the sickness in their herd they would need to "bleed the cows"—rancher-speak for doing a blood test. They drew blood from a number of cows and took the vials of blood to their vet for testing. The results showed that the cows were dangerously deficient in a number of essential minerals that cows normally get from grazing. So Lori and her husband started a mineral feeding program. I asked how they applied the minerals to the cows, and she said: "We just put them out in buckets, and the cows gravitated toward the minerals and started licking—they seemed to know what they needed. At first, we couldn't believe how much they ate or how fast they were using up the minerals, but then the cows seemed to grow satiated, or maybe their mineral levels balanced, because they consumed smaller amounts. Our neighbors thought we were crazy—but our cows grew healthy."

After a short time, the herd's health improved dramatically, calves were born healthy and gained the proper weight, and there were no more calves in the kitchen on IVs. Lori also learned the root cause of the mineral deficit in her herd: geologic evidence, such as a lack of glacial polish on the rocks in the area, revealed that the glaciers that had tilled the surface of the Great Plains during the last ice age had not passed over a 50-mile-wide swath of land where Lori's ranch was located—so the soil was not as rich with minerals churned up from the glacial action of ice turning stone to dust. Before they retired and sold their ranch, Lori and her husband continued their mineral supplement program and consistently had healthier calves and cows than their ranching neighbors—and needed no drugs.

Lori remembered that when the new owner took over the ranch and she told him about their mineral supplement program, "he just shook his head, laughed, and said, 'Pshaww.' Within a year he was injecting calves with drugs to keep them alive, and once their systems are damaged they never grow as big or healthy. I was amazed how fast they got sick again when the new owner stopped the mineral supplements."

The lessons in Lori's story and the striking parallels to what I do in my practice left me speechless. Even though Lori's cows were given the same food as other cows all across the region, the particular environment these cows were raised in resulted in browse that lacked minerals essential to their health and deprived Lori's herd of critical sustenance. Most ranchers in the area dealt with the problem by treating the cows' symptoms of ill health with drugs, but because the drugs didn't get to the root of the problem, they didn't see the same quality of results as Lori had obtained by correcting the cows' core imbalances.

To uncover the core problem in their herd and determine what was out of balance, Lori and her husband tested the animals' blood. This is essentially what I do every day in my clinic. Moreover, there are parallels between the unwillingness of the new owner to take their solution seriously and mainstream medicine's cynical view of the functional medicine I practice. I've been called the "Witch Doctor from Wilson" by physicians in the area, and when I speak to traditionally trained physicians about my solutions, I am met with a cool quiet at best, and at worst outright disapproval. In another parallel, Lori, looking "outside the box" for a better solution to her cows' woes than just giving them drugs, asked the local vet to apply laboratory technology to test the cows' blood, and then, with what she learned from the results, kept the herd healthy for many years using nutrition, not IV therapies, drugs, or antibiotics. And just as I try to help my patients get to a point where they don't need me anymore, Lori didn't need her vet anymore once she found her solution.

For you, dear reader, the parallel is that you may not be able to prevent or reverse heart disease entirely on your own, although your own effort is critical no matter what kind of advanced medicine your solution includes. Many of my patients benefit greatly from the deep insights into systemic imbalance and inflammation provided by modern blood tests. The great thing is that you were born at the right time. These tests are now far more affordable than they were just a few years ago, and a number of them are even covered by insurance programs because they are considered "preventative." Indeed they are. And once you know what your system needs, you can manage your internal balance for decades—just as Lori did for her cows—without ongoing drugs or expensive medical treatment.

To help you understand the intimidating and overwhelming results of modern blood tests, this next section will give you the same information I give my patients so that they can interpret the results of blood tests.

By the way, Lori is now in her early seventies, the only drug she takes is a half-dose of her blood pressure medication every day, and she has healthy cholesterol levels. She told me, as she pushed the croutons to the side of her salad that day we had lunch, "I feel way better than I did when I was fifty-five. With such good health at my age, every day is Christmas."

Looking Inside

When you think about working with a doctor, take a lesson from Lori and her cows. The vet didn't tell Lori what to do, but rather, when she asked for help, assisted her in taking a closer look at the imbalances that were ailing her herd. Then Lori herself delivered the medicine (in the form of mineral supplements, not drugs) and maintained the health of the herd without the vet.

Blood tests provide an incredible view of our inner workings on a molecular scale, and they can play a critical role in optimizing your solution for your particular body. I regularly give the following blood tests to my patients and recommend them for anyone who wants to improve her heart health:

- Food sensitivity/intolerance tests

- Heart panel: Consists of a lipid profile (cholesterol) with particle size for individual risk, blood sugar and insulin levels, and inflammatory markers

- Thyroid and hormone function tests

In my clinic, the results of these tests are then layered on top of the patient's story, family history, personal goals, a combination of my own and the patient's intuition, and other factors revealed by the Heart Solution Matrix. We then use this combination of insights and data to further refine her solution, which may or may not involve drugs—and often involves getting off medication prescribed by other physicians, or at least lowering the doses.

According to a Mayo Clinic study, about half the population of the United States is on two prescription medications, and 20 percent take at least five. More women than men receive prescription medications, and get this: almost one-quarter of American women between fifty and sixty-four are prescribed antidepressants. Additionally, almost one-third of Americans over forty are prescribed statin drugs to lower their cholesterol and to, at least in theory, protect their hearts. (By now you know that for you as an individual the chance of statins saving your life from heart disease is very small.)

You may very well benefit from prescription medicine, but in my opinion and experience, we are currently facing an epidemic of vast and overzealous use of pharmaceuticals, and it is extremely likely that you don't need the medicine your doctor has prescribed to you. Additionally, there's a good chance the medicine you're taking may be doing you more harm than good. Most of my patients do better replacing pharmaceuticals with the therapies and lifestyle changes recommended in this book and by other holistic, lifestyle medicine programs. And I'm not alone—even the CDC has listed practicing healthy living habits as the number-one method to prevent heart disease. The US government recommends a trial of therapeutic life-style changes for six weeks as *first-line therapy* for elevated choles-terol and blood sugar prior to reaching for any drug. Data specific to women from research into the Mediterranean diet show that the diet alone may decrease the risk of death by any cause by over 50 per-cent, whereas statin drugs have never shown more than a 30 percent benefit for any group. For the risk of death from heart disease specifi-cally, adherence to the Mediterranean diet may lower risk by about the same amount as statin drugs. Studies into the diet are under scrutiny, but the trend is clear—lifestyle medicine rivals or beats drugs when it comes to chronic disease treatment. Add the other elements of the Heart Solution for Women and the program you're probably brewing in your mind by this point will do far more to heal your heart and save your life than any drug.

I can't recommend that you stop taking the drugs that you're on without seeing you, but what I can do is explain the process and tests I use to help people develop a Precision, Personalized Solution with minimal and extremely conservative application of pharmaceuticals. If you're not currently taking drugs but at some point your doctor suggests that you start, I can also recommend that you gather as much information as possible and try other methods first. And if you are on medication, ask your doctor to help you reduce, optimize, or even eliminate your dose of prescription medication or over-the-counter pharmaceuticals. To help you progress toward this goal, this final chapter will share the tests I use and some natural alternatives to the most common medications I see people taking. I'll also describe the steps I take to help my patients reduce, optimize, or eliminate their use of drugs.

You can follow almost every recommendation in this book on your own, but you'll need to enlist your doctor's help to get a modern blood test, which is an incredible way to learn what will benefit your heart the most. The main hurdle to get past is the tendency of most American doctors to use old-fashioned "health fair"–style testing, which looks at such basic parameters that you learn nothing about your personal risk or what you can do about it. There's far better testing out there if you know what to ask for.

Food Sensitivity/Intolerance Testing

The blood test for food sensitivities or food intolerances does not look for severe allergic reactions like the peanut or shellfish allergies we're all familiar with. Food sensitivities and intolerances can take days to develop and weeks to go away, and they are difficult to figure out on your own, even with an elimination diet. This blood test is one of the cornerstones of functional medicine and has been integral to helping millions of functional medicine patients around the world go from a life of disease to a life of vitality. For you, the food sensitivity test may reveal that one (or several) of the foods you consume on a near-daily basis are poison to your body. The food sensitivity blood test is inexpensive, can be done through a finger prick and a few drops of blood, is readily available through your family physician, and provides an incredible insight into your particular body.

The results of any food sensitivity test should be confirmed via elimination testing because the tests are not 100 percent accurate and false positives are common. If my client's test shows numerous high-level reactions to a diverse range of nutrient-rich foods, we follow a careful elimination protocol to determine which foods are indeed causing an inflammatory reaction in her body and which are either false positives or only minor irritations. This elimination process usually goes something like this:

1. Eliminate the foods showing the highest reactions for one month.

2. Supplement with nutrient smoothies made with pure, non-GMO, plant-based (not whey-, gluten-, or soy-based) proteins that provide the same nutrition as the eliminated food. For example, if a patient shows a dairy sensitivity, we supplement with protein smoothies and calcium to ensure that she receives adequate nutrition.

3. After one month, add the most missed food back into your diet in small amounts and monitor yourself for symptoms of food sensitivity using the 7-Day Food Log (see Appendix). It may take twenty-four to forty-eight hours for the symptoms to show. Keep in mind that usually only one in ten symptoms will be digestive (bloating, fullness, heartburn, diarrhea, constipation). Other possible symptoms are migraine, fatigue, PMS, mood changes, skin changes or rash, and insomnia.

4. Continue following these steps with each food until you find the culprit. Then continue to avoid that food and replace its

nutrition with alternative food sources and supplemental nutrition if needed.

As you can see, using the elimination approach without a blood test would take a lengthy and scientific self-assessment that few of us are ready to handle. A blood test is easier, more accurate, faster, and relatively inexpensive, costing from $150 to $300 depending on the specific test.

The most amazing thing about food sensitivity testing is that once you know what foods are causing your problems, *you will eventually stop craving them.* In fact, not only will you find it easy to turn them down, but you may start looking at those foods with revulsion. I know this from experience and from watching my patients discover the foods that are poisoning them. This reaction is partly psychological and partly physiological: your body knows well what is good for it, and once you break the habit of consuming a food that is poisoning you, your body quickly develops an aversion to it.

Direct Measurement Cholesterol Test/Heart Panel

This is the test that should be the normal test of heart health, not the health fair–style cholesterol score that we're all familiar with. The heart panel we use in the Meno Clinic Center for Functional Medicine to test for heart disease risk is the most advanced testing available. Our test will break down your cholesterol into its heart-healing and heart-damaging elements—not just the total cholesterol. This includes your levels of the dangerous cholesterol particles such as bad LDL, sticky triglycerides as well as good, fluffy HDL cholesterol. We also assess the particles that are part of the more advanced cholesterol profile that further individualize your risk—small dense LDL, apolipoprotein A and B, lipoprotein A. This reveals the inflammatory fireballs that show who is most at risk and provide early detection of who may have a heart attack soon. This information not only is predictive of heart disease risk, but also allows us to track the reduction of risk and cooling of inflammation as they follow their Precision, Personalized Solution.

In addition, the test looks at the hormone balance of your symphony, including insulin, blood sugar, and other metabolic imbalances as well as thyroid, adrenal, and female hormone health; blood pressure dysfunction indicators that predict future blood pressure problems; and the critical and actionable vitamin and mineral levels, including the heart-repairing ones we've talked about: folate, vitamin B12, coenzyme Q_{10}, omega-3, vitamin D, calcium, magnesium, and potassium. We also test your genetics to complete the precision, personalized assessment of *your* risk to prevent and reverse heart disease.

Providing the perfect assessment tool to use in conjunction with your own intuitive insight into your health, the heart panel allows you to develop your solution with greatly increased precision. You can use the results, combined with your doctor's evaluation of those results, to determine which supplements, at what dose, could help you and whether you need pharmaceuticals. The heart panel results also give you an excellent baseline from which to track your progress in your quest for heart health and overall vitality.

If the results put up flags for dangerously high or low levels of any of the biomarkers measured in the panel, the next step is to apply your own Precision, Personalized Solution for three to six months before taking the test again. It is in the second taking of the test that I see my patients attain Wonder Woman levels of discipline and motivation. When you see a very specific and real measurement of a particular indicator of heart health improve for the better because of your own actions, the power of individualized medicine becomes yours for the taking and inspires good decision-making for long into the future. As an added motivator, improvements in the heart panel are usually accompanied by greater vitality and energy, better sleep and mood, and improved physical presence. One of my favorite parts of the follow-up appointment is a patient's report that her friends are saying, "You look great!" or "How did you lose that weight?" or "Why is your skin so clear?" or "How did your hair get so full?" I'm not kidding. The pleasant unintended consequences of improved heart health are incredible.

Unfortunately, most doctors are still not taking advantage of these new advances in laboratory testing for heart disease risk. I teach thousands of doctors each year, and many of them have not even heard of these cutting-edge tests that are available to all of their patients. And that's a big part of the problem: there are lots of great doctors out there, but they have not been given the right tools to identify *your* personal risk and prevent heart disease for *you*.

Now we do have those tools, though, so ask your doctor to help you take and then interpret these tests. The following guidelines to the inflammatory markers of the heart panel will give you the information you need to ask your doctor the right questions (and make your doctor do her or his homework to give you good answers).

High-sensitivity C-reactive protein (HS-CRP)

C-reactive protein (CRP) is made by the liver in response to inflammation and infection, and the part called HS-CRP (high-sensitivity CRP) used for the heart assessment was found twenty-five years ago to be an independent marker of heart disease risk. If this number is elevated, you are much more likely to have a heart attack sometime in the future. The usual interpretation of the HS-CRP level focuses on heart inflammation, but it really is an indicator of inflammation throughout the body. Several studies have shown it to be a risk independent from cholesterol. Pharmaceutical companies are now jumping on the CRP bandwagon, so you will see medications targeting CRP coming soon.

Lipoprotein-associated phospholipase A2 (PLAC2)

Two tests developed in the last few years that are now part of the heart panel are far more sensitive and predictive of your current risk than anything we've had before. These new markers are myeloperoxidase (MPO) and lipoprotein-associated phospholipase A2 (LP-PLA2), or what we call PLAC2. These measurements of the intensity of the fire inside your heart tell you how much risk you have for a plaque to rupture and cause a heart attack today. But remember: as with all the biomarkers measured in a heart panel, you can manipulate these two with lifestyle medicine.

The PLAC2 is a result of your body trying to get rid of those small, sticky cholesterol marbles that are trying to make heart blood vessel plaque, and it fans the flames of inflammation in doing so. The PLAC2 level reveals how many of those small sticky marbles are trying to make plaque and, more importantly, how much inflammation is brewing in the plaque. We all have plaques, both large and small, and they can be either very stable, with a thick "cap" that keeps them from rupturing, or thin and fragile and prone to rupture. The measurement of PLAC2 (and MPO) gives you an idea of how much inflammation is chewing away at that plaque and making it thinner and more likely to rupture. If the plaque does rupture, your body will respond to the ensuing firestorm by forming a blood clot, which can completely block the flow of blood. When the blood clot blocks blood flow to the heart, you have a heart attack; when the blood clot blocks blood flow to your brain, you have a stroke. PLAC2 is a way to assess the state of the plaques in your arteries.

Myeloperoxidase (MPO)

MPO is an enzyme released by the immune system that can be measured to assess your body's response to damaged heart blood vessels that have become thin and unstable due to accumulation of the small, sticky cholesterol marbles under the plaque and the inflammation eating away at the plaque that could make it rupture.

When those small, sticky marbles enter the blood vessels of your heart, your body tries to remove them by recruiting the immune system to send in immune warrior cells. These warriors wrongly think the small, sticky cholesterol particles are bacteria or viruses that have invaded the body. The warriors release MPO, but instead of killing the cholesterol the warriors have mistaken for a virus or bacteria, the MPO creates a special confusion in the plaque by making a "foamy cell." This is actually a cell of the immune system full of bleach-like cholesterol that looks like soapy bubbles. It acts like lava bubbling under a volcano: it wants to burst through the heart artery wall, and if this happens, your body responds by creating a blood clot, leading to heart attack or stroke. Traditional blood tests like the calculated cholesterol test and even the stress tests and angiograms given by cardiologists will not be able to see elevated MPO levels, but the right blood tests will.

We are entering a new era of heart disease risk assessment and treatment. At long last, we have tools that reveal the specifics of your risk, but it is unlikely that your doctor will suggest that you take these tests unless you ask for them. The typical doctor's response to why we don't test everyone for biomarkers like HS-CRP and MPO is "Well, there really isn't anything we can do about it, so why bother testing for them."

What they mean when they say, "There really isn't anything we can do about it" is that *there are no drugs to change these biomarkers*, but in my clinic I see lifestyle medicine improve these biomarkers all the time.

How to Get Off Pharmaceuticals

The most effective and safest way to find the optimal dose of a prescription medication, reduce your dose, or better yet stop taking it entirely is to slowly reduce your dose while simultaneously replacing it with natural or lifestyle medicine measures. Going cold turkey can be dangerous and usually doesn't work.

If at all possible, you should reduce or get off medication under physician supervision. Most likely, your physician will not be supportive of this goal of reducing your medication. If that's the case, tell your doctor: "I don't think the medication is serving me well, and I want to try reducing my dose while investigating some other options that might work better for me in the long run. I am willing to do my part by making some lifestyle changes with better food choices and exercise."

The physician's role should then be to monitor your progress to make sure you're safely changing your therapy from pharmaceutical-based to nutrition- and lifestyle-based. If your physician refuses, find another physician. It is possible that you will be best served by a combination of pharmaceuticals and lifestyle medicine, but I can say with confidence that most of the pharmaceuticals being taken today are not solving the individual's core problem, and a great many of them are making matters worse rather than better. And the bottom line on drugs as they relate to heart health is that, if they are not solving your core problem, they are increasing your risk in the long run by preventing you from finding your solution.

In the following section, I present some of the most common pharmaceuticals that have proven detrimental to heart health on an individual level. I also give you recommendations for alternative treatment, as well as questions to ask your doctor when enlisting her or his help to avoid, minimize, or cease the use of pharmaceuticals.

Antibiotics

Ask this question when your doctor suggests antibiotics:

Are you sure I have a bacterial infection and not a virus?

If you get a bacterial infection, antibiotics may save your life. But just because you're sick doesn't mean you need antibiotics. If you get a cold, bronchitis, or other viral infection, taking antibiotics will not only fail to make you better but destroy your helpful gut bacteria, increasing your risk of leaky gut, and add to the general increase in antibiotic resistance and the development of superbugs that cannot be treated with current antibiotics. The CDC estimates that as much as one half of all antibiotic use is unnecessary and that every year doctors in the United States write 47 million unnecessary prescriptions for antibiotics.

If you must take antibiotics, add prebiotic and probiotic treatment to rehabilitate your microbiome, but a word of caution: never take a probiotic and an antibiotic at the same time of day or they will effectively cancel each other out! You must separate the timing by several hours. This is crucial because if you need an antibiotic for infection, you really want it to work. Most antibiotics are taken twice a day, so take the antibiotic with breakfast and dinner and the probiotic with lunch. If in doubt, wait to start your probiotics until after you've completed the course of antibiotics.

A lot of advertising hype suggests that a product with billions and billions of probiotic colonies is better. More is not always better—the quality and stability of the probiotic are much more important than the high counts claimed on the bottle. Quality is queen.

Prebiotics are simply the foods you eat that feed those good girl probiotics and nurture the crazy complex microbiome jungle living in your gut. Good food sources of prebiotics include leeks, onions, garlic, asparagus, dandelion greens, Jerusalem artichoke, and similar vegetables. Though best eaten raw for optimal prebiotic effect, these veggies can be cooked and still retain some prebiotic benefit.

Nonsteroidal Anti-Inflammatory Drugs

The question to ask when your doctor suggests nonsteroidal anti-inflammatory drugs (NSAIDs) is:

If I don't take the anti-inflammatories, will I still heal the same in the long run?

If you'll heal without the drug, then don't take it. In the vast majority of cases, NSAIDs don't do anything that your body wouldn't do naturally on its own. The symptoms may not disappear as quickly as they would if you popped pills, but the end result will be better and your body will thank you for it.

Also bear in mind that if you're that canary in the coal mine of sensitivity, taking NSAIDs could put you in the hospital or even kill you. It's been estimated that each year more than 100,000 people are hospitalized due to NSAID-related gastrointestinal problems and that over 16,000 people die from these complications. NSAIDs are also the number-two cause of leaky gut developing (antibiotics are number one), because NSAIDs disrupt the gut lining and start you down that road to leaky gut inflammation. Also consider this: many orthopedic surgeons forbid NSAID use after surgery because they can impede the healing process.

ALTERNATIVES TO NSAIDS

- Rest

- If the pain is in the joints, ice the inflamed area for the first seventy-two hours

- Green leafy vegetables, blueberries, beets, turmeric, ginger, salmon, nuts, broccoli, flax seeds

- Consider a trial of avoiding nightshade vegetables

- Removal of the root cause of inflammation through lifestyle and nutrition

SUPPLEMENT ALTERNATIVES TO NSAIDS

- Theramine, an amino acid blend known as a "medical food," requires a physician prescription. It has been proven to be as effective as naproxen (which used to require a prescription) for treating pain and reducing inflammation and comes without the damaging side effects.

- Wobenzyme is an enzyme-based natural product used as the number-one anti-inflammatory in Germany, preferred over any medication.

- Zyflamend, an herbal blend based on holy basil and used for inflammation and pain reduction, has also been shown to kill cancer cells in the lab.

- Omega-3 fish oil can be effective taken at a high dose of 3–4 grams per day.

- Cannabidiol (CBD) oil is an emerging supplement with promising potential. The medical version has no tetrahydrocannabinol (THC), the psychoactive ingredient in marijuana, and there are more receptors in your brain for this cannabinoid compound than for any other neurotransmitter.

Antidepressants

Ask your doctor:

Can you help me fix my thyroid and hormone balance before you put me on antidepressants?

Is this really true depression or is it a less severe imbalance?

Is my thyroid working optimally?

Is my vitamin D level optimal for me?

Can you help me try some lifestyle medicine and supplement support first?

The problem with antidepressants is that they do nothing to solve the root problem causing the depression. Some studies have shown that the drugs result in a reduction in suicide, but among women ages thirty to seventy-five, antidepressant drug use does not change the suicide rate. Additionally, antidepressant medicine can increase the risk of suicide for some people—and you may be one of them. This potentially fatal side effect is common enough that the FDA requires a black box warning for suicidality associated with antidepressants. Also, the National Institute of Mental Health's famous STAR*D (Sequenced Treatment Alternatives to Relieve Depression) trial showed that after three months of treatment, two-thirds of patients had received no benefit at all from antidepressant use.

There are now genetic tests available that look at the specific reasons why you may have depression, and we use them in my clinic. These tests can help you decide which medication may actually work for your particular genetics, but they also reveal insights into where your serotonin system is broken. You are then better able to use natural supplements to support and repair the deficiency and resolve your depression without drugs.

ALTERNATIVES TO ANTIDEPRESSANTS

- Lifestyle medicine

- Exercise—in some studies, thirty minutes of aerobic exercise daily outperformed antidepressants

- Exercise in groups for the social benefits

- Optimization of adrenal, thyroid, and female hormones

- Optimization of blood sugar to prevent dramatic highs and lows in energy to the brain

- Exposure to direct daylight or a light therapy lamp (which must be 10,000 lux strength)

- Eliminate caffeine (can cause desensitization to serotonin)

- Stop taking statin drugs

SUPPLEMENT ALTERNATIVES TO ANTIDEPRESSANTS

- 5-hydroxytryptophan (5-HTP)—an amino acid proven to improve sleep, mood, and serotonin (*dose:* typically 50–100 milligrams once or twice per day, preferably at bedtime to promote sleep)

- S-adenosylmethionine (SAM-e) (*dose:* 200–600 micrograms, taken in the morning)

- St. John's wort (works especially well in younger women, but beware: it can make birth control ineffective!)

- Vitamin D

- Magnesium

- B vitamins

- Several other promising natural therapies, including a lavender-based supplement

Osteoporosis Drugs

Questions to ask your doctor:

Why do I have osteoporosis and can you help me remove the underlying cause?

What are the risks of the medications?

Do you know about N-terminal telopeptide (NTx) testing to assess actual bone physiology?

Osteoporosis costs Americans $16 billion each year and affects 200 million women worldwide and it's been estimated that as many as 80 percent of osteoporosis fractures go unreported. We don't typically think of osteoporosis as related to heart health, but everything is related in the human body, and emerging evidence shows a strong association between heart disease and bone health. The relationship is complex and much is still unknown, but the data show that as bone mineral density decreases, heart disease increases. In women specifically, osteoporosis is a strong predictor of heart disease.

And that's where the drugs come in. If you're taking drugs for osteoporosis, you're not solving the problem. Even worse, on rare occasions people who take osteoporosis drugs suffer from bone death, usually in the jaw and thigh bones. In these instances, drugs can cause the exact bone decay we're trying to prevent. The best way to prevent osteoporosis is to start a lifestyle that supports bone health as early in life as possible. This is easy because it's the same lifestyle you'll be living anyway to take care of your heart!

I also see women who've been put on a medication for osteoporosis because, even though their hip density is fantastic, their lower back shows osteoporosis. However, any DEXA testing results that indicate osteoporosis in the lower back can be thrown off by a history of back injury or slight lower back curvature. Additionally, the DEXA bone density scan is typically covered by insurance only every two years, is expensive, has a low radiation dose, and does not tell you what you really want to know: *Am I making stronger bones right now?*

Instead, ask for an NTx test—an inexpensive urine test that assesses, in real time, the balance between the cells in your body building bone and those that are tearing it down.

ALTERNATIVES TO OSTEOPOROSIS DRUGS

- Increase fruit and vegetable consumption

- Sustain physical activity throughout life

- Increase back muscle strength

- Reduce time spent sitting

- Avoid moderate or heavy alcohol consumption (low or none is better)

- Stop smoking

- Avoid corticosteroids, antidepressants, sedatives, and anti-anxiety medications

- Optimize protein absorption

- Take apple cider vinegar daily

- Increase weight-bearing exercise—but do it safely!

SUPPLEMENT ALTERNATIVES TO OSTEOPOROSIS DRUGS

- Strontium anecdotally has demonstrated amazing results in my patients, and its effectiveness has been proven in several studies.

- Calcium is controversial—there are big arguments over types of calcium, as several kinds exist—but what matters most is quality. Grocery store calcium just doesn't cut it. I typically recommend 800–1,200 milligrams, but don't take calcium supplements unless you know you are deficient in calcium.

- Sublingual vitamin D can be taken for optimal absorption (a blood level of 80 ng/ml). See Chapter 8 for dose. Vitamin K2 is added to most high-quality brands for optimal effectiveness.

- Protein smoothies and healthy protein sources are good not only for your heart but for your bones as well.

Proton Pump Inhibitors/Acid-Blocking Medicines

Questions to ask your doctor:

Do you think my heartburn is caused by too little or too much acid? (Best answer: "It could be either.")

What do you suggest I try before taking drugs?

Proton pump inhibitors (PPIs) sound like something that would be used aboard the starship *Enterprise,* but in reality they are a common medication used for heartburn and intestinal discomfort that increases the risk of dementia, osteoporosis, kidney disease, and other problems—including a staggering 25 percent increase in chance of death. Some PPIs are available over the counter and are used by millions of people for durations of time that were never approved.

One of the first things I hear from my patients who take PPIs is that the box says to take it for only fourteen days, but as soon as they stopped taking the PPI their heartburn got worse because they had even more acid. So they started taking the PPI again, even though the fourteen-day warning scared them. Marketing genius.

As far as heart health goes, PPI medications increase oxidative stress and damage endothelial cells, those critical barriers lining the arteries. These medications include aspirin, omeprazole, and a handful of other meds ending in "-prazole," as well as the brand names Prilosec, Prevacid, Dexilant, AcipHex, and Protonix.

People take PPI medicine primarily to reduce stomach acid production, but these drugs don't even work very well to treat the symptoms they're designed to reduce. PPI medication is a perfect example of the worst of pharmaceuticals at work—treating the symptom rather than the cause, with potential side effects that you wouldn't wish on your worst enemy. And ironically, many cases of stomach upset are caused by the side effects of other medications—people are taking PPI drugs to help them endure the side effects of other drugs. Remember that story about the old woman who swallowed a spider to catch the fly?

Naturopathic doctors typically attribute heartburn issues to too little stomach acid, and mainstream medical doctors typically attribute it to too much acid. Which view is right? Neither.

The correct answer is that heartburn can be caused by *either* too much or too little stomach acid, and there is no one solution for everyone. I've seen "natural" doctors tell patients to count betaine hydrochloric acid tablets as they take them one by one until they feel a burning sensation, subtract one from the total, and take that many with each meal. Their patients end up taking somewhere around six pills with every meal. That's crazy, if you ask me.

For heartburn, I try to use food as medicine and supplement only when necessary. If you have a history of ulcer disease, you should never take PPIs without doctor supervision.

ALTERNATIVES TO PPI DRUGS

- Apple cider vinegar—I know, this recommendation seems counterintuitive because vinegar is acidic, but apple cider vinegar lowers acidity as well as blood sugar and blood pressure, and it promotes detoxification. Drink two tablespoons as a shot before each meal, or through a straw so as to not damage the enamel on your teeth when drinking it long-term.

- Baking soda—One teaspoon in a glass of water can sometimes help as much as a PPI drug, and it's safe.

- Ginger—My favorite heartburn remedy is to add a few slices of ginger to hot water and let it steep for twenty minutes before drinking.

- Drink chamomile tea.

- Stop smoking.

- Don't lie down immediately after eating.

- Eat smaller portions and more frequent meals.

- Eat more fermented vegetables.

- Don't eat nightshade vegetables (such as tomatoes, peppers, and eggplant).

SUPPLEMENT ALTERNATIVES TO PPI DRUGS

- Glutamine—As it is one of my favorite supplements, I use glutamine in combination with zinc carnosine. The best form of it is powder mixed in water, but capsules work too. Cancer patients should discuss glutamine with their physician before taking the supplement. The usual dose is 3–5 grams per day.

- Zinc carnosine—This supplement has been proven equal to several PPI medications in multiple trials. The dose is typically 75 milligrams per day.

- Betaine—This supplement comes in a variety of doses and must be used with caution if you have a history of ulcers because there is usually hydrochloric acid in it.

- Plant-based digestive enzymes may relieve heartburn.

Cholesterol Drugs

Statins, or cholesterol-lowering drugs, are front and center in the discussion on heart health. We already talked about them in depth in Chapter 2, but we haven't talked about when to take them or how to get off of them if you don't truly benefit from them. I prescribe statins for some patients, but I've also gotten many more people—hundreds of them—off of statin drugs by prescribing supplements, lifestyle, and diet. Off statins, you're far better situated to prevent heart disease than if you're on them, unable to properly monitor your vascular health, and facing their side effects, which, as mentioned earlier, include muscle damage and an increased risk of diabetes.

I was recently lecturing in Ireland, and one of the other lectures I heard was by one of the United Kingdom's leading cardiologists, who explained that basically no one benefits from a statin drug. "No one" were his exact words. He also claimed that we have created the largest vitamin deficiency ever seen on the planet—a depletion of coenzyme Q_{10}—by using statins.

When researchers first looked for a way to reduce cholesterol through drugs, they decided to build on the chemical framework of red yeast rice extract, which acts as a natural statin to lower cholesterol, improve circulation, and alleviate digestive problems. The extract itself remains a powerful and popular supplement for reducing cholesterol levels and reversing heart disease. In my opinion, unless you're in the extremely high-risk category for heart disease or have already suffered a heart attack or stroke, red yeast rice is a better option than statin drugs if you have dangerously high cholesterol.

In my practice, I use both the drug and the extract, but I prefer prescribing red yeast rice when possible because of its added benefits: fatty acids, somewhat less severe side effects and risk in stopping its use. Red yeast rice and statin drugs can have similar side effects, including reduced CoQ_{10} levels, which can cause muscle and liver damage, so I include CoQ_{10} supplements with both red yeast rice and statin prescriptions.

Statins also encapsulate perfectly one of the problems with modern evidence-based medicine: only the positive "evidence" for medications is commonly published and negative "evidence" is often not reported. The US Congress requires that drugs—but not supplements—be tested for safety and efficacy, but it does not require that study results be published promptly. This massive loophole allows pharmaceutical companies to use and publish the data of their choice. For example, in 2004 an article appeared in the *Journal of the American Medical Association* (*JAMA*) about how well the statin simvastatin worked. It reported that the drug causes muscle damage in 8 out of 10,000 patients—one out of every 1,250 people. In 2011, seven years later, it was revealed that this same simvastatin research from 2004 showed muscle damage in 61 of 1,000 patients—about 1 out of every 16 people. Either the data was interpreted wrong to start with, or the definition of "muscle damage" was conveniently adjusted to make the drug look less harmful, or it was an example of a situation where negative results were not published. Regardless of the reason, this incredible result, one potentially damaging to the multibillion-dollar statin market, was not reported for seven years!

After the seven-years-too-late release of the full simvastatin study, Europe banned 80-milligram doses of simvastatin, but it is still prescribed in the United States to this day. Muscle poisoning from high-dose simvastatin is an all-too-common story in my clinic. I recently had a client from Tennessee who came to Jackson Hole for a consult. She was tired all the time. She had low CoQ_{10}, which caused mitochondria poisoning in her muscles. Her liver test was elevated, which means that her detox system wasn't functioning, and her test for the muscle enzyme creatine phosphokinase (CPK) was elevated, indicating poisoning and breakdown of muscle tissue. She was taking the 80-milligram simvastatin dose. No wonder she was pissed off when I told her about the data on simvastatin muscle damage and Europe's ban on the dose she was taking. We got her off the 80-milligram simvastatin, and her symptoms improved dramatically.

For people on statins, I follow the recommendation of my friend Stephen Sinatra, a renowned cardiologist. Everyone on a statin should consider this: To minimize and recover from muscle damage from a statin, take 100–200 milligrams of high-quality CoQ_{10}, 5 grams of ribose, and 200 milligrams of carnitine daily. Double those doses if you have existing muscle damage or fatigue. An example of how well this formula works is a Stanford professor who had always biked to work, 20 miles every day. After taking statins, he got to the point where he could barely walk up a flight of stairs. He had seen multiple doctors for over a year, without success, even though he stopped taking the statin. He flew out to see me for a consultation, we gave him a triple dose of this formula, and within six months he was back to biking to work again.

Simvastatin now comes with an FDA warning label—the ubiquitous black box—informing users about its dangers to the liver and muscles as well as the increased risk of diabetes and dementia it carries. To lower the average person's cholesterol with a pill, we're increasing many individuals' risk of heart disease. See the conflict here?

When I prescribe statin drugs, I work out the plan with each client carefully to minimize side effects and maximize benefits. I also choose the long-acting statins that can be taken every other day or two to three times a week; they deliver the same benefit with many fewer side effects and less risk.

I believe that statins are an excellent medicine for the very narrow group of people who benefit from them. The problem with statin use is that we're not looking at the risk equation of using them properly. Consider the way mountaineers view risk. A mountaineer who summited K2, the world's second-highest mountain and one of the deadliest, explained risk with this equation:

$$Risk = Probability \times Consequences$$

In other words, if a mountaineer is climbing on a cliff of solid rock, there is a risk of a rock falling off the top and hitting her or him. The consequence of that would be high, but the probability is extremely low, making this an acceptable risk for most mountaineers. On the other hand, getting struck by lightning while standing on the top of a large rock spire in a thunderstorm has not only high consequence but also relatively high probability. The smart mountaineer avoids standing on summits in lightning storms.

Applying this definition of risk to the world of medicine, when I prescribe statins (or any other drugs or supplements for that matter), I look at the consequences for the patient of not having the medicine.

If her heart health is really poor, the probability of her having a heart attack or stroke is so high that the potential negative consequences of taking the drug are relatively low. Therefore, the overall added risk of her taking the statin drug is low.

On the other hand, for a patient who has slightly reduced vascular function and high cholesterol, eats a terrible diet, and doesn't exercise, the equation is very different. There is a good chance that lifestyle changes will reduce this patient's risk of heart disease. According to the NNT evaluation of statins (see Chapter 2), the probability that putting her on statins will help her is very low, and doing so could also have very high consequences—not only physical side effects like diabetes and muscle damage but also the "licensing effect" (feeling liberated from making sound decisions about your health because you're taking medicine). The risk of putting this kind of patient on statin drugs is too high, and I will try numerous other treatments before resorting to drugs.

Obviously, the risk evaluation equation for medicine is complex. But by looking at the probability and consequences of your decision-making, you're well ahead of the vast majority of people on statin drugs—as well as many of the doctors prescribing them. Statin drugs also have an anti-inflammatory effect, which has a lot to do with their efficacy. However, there are safer ways to reduce cholesterol and inflammation in your body than taking cholesterol-lowering medication.

Being told by a doctor that you need statin drugs is a strong indicator that your heart needs more help than statin drugs alone can fix. Think of it this way: the majority of patients given statin drugs for life are accepting an unhealthy vascular system in the hope that the drugs will protect them from heart disease, but they fail to recognize that obscuring the symptoms of vascular disease with drugs could have potentially severe consequences in the future, as well as side effects that will decrease their quality of life in the present.

Most patients with heart disease risk who take the functional medicine approach and use lifestyle and diet changes to treat their vascular health end up with a much healthier vascular system than patients who rely on statin drugs. Many people who take statin drugs continue their dietary and lifestyle assault on their heart and the rest of their vascular system even as their cholesterol numbers improve. Statins are a little like cheating on a test—your score may be good, but you really didn't benefit from the lesson.

Getting off of Statin Drugs

As I'm sure you're already thinking, it's better to try every safe non-pharmaceutical recommendation in this book—and in every other book written about heart health—to see if you can heal your heart without statin drugs before you let your doctor put you on a prescription for life.

Once you're taking statins, you'll find it very difficult to find a doctor who will encourage you to get off of them. But if you insist, a good doctor should be willing to help you monitor your progress in reducing your dose as you gradually replace the drug with lifestyle therapies. There is a very real risk to stopping statin use, particularly for people who have been using them for many years. After quitting statins cold turkey, cholesterol and the inflammatory C-reactive protein (CRP) both increase rapidly. It's almost as if your body becomes "addicted" to the drug. Even so, one in five people who start taking statins decide to stop, most of them without a plan for doing so safely. If you decide to stop taking statins, do it safely, with doctor supervision.

Getting off statins requires careful monitoring of cholesterol levels as well as a sustained and disciplined increase in lifestyle medicine and heart-protecting supplements to replace the statin's cholesterol-lowering power. The trifecta of supplements I use to replace statins is red yeast rice extract, niacin, and omega-3.

Red Yeast Rice Extract

Modern statin drugs are based on red yeast rice extract, a monacolin extract and ancient Chinese heart tonic. This natural statin blocks cholesterol production just as all synthetic statins do but is much less toxic.

If you are considering supplements of any kind, I recommend that you check out the Consumer Lab website (www.consumerlab.com) to determine the quality and ingredients. When Consumer Lab looked at ten over-the-counter red yeast rice products, they found toxins in eight of them. Statins and red yeast rice extract share both risks and benefits: they are both medicines that should be taken only as part of a professionally managed plan to achieve optimal vascular health.

When used in combination with fish oil and lifestyle therapies, red yeast rice extract matches or exceeds statins' cholesterol-lowering power, and it has the added benefit of reducing triglyceride levels, which statin drugs do not do. For heart health—and every other kind of health for that matter—the therapy of red yeast rice and fish oil combined with lifestyle medicine is far superior to statins. Statin therapy does one thing—lower cholesterol levels—and does it really well. The therapy outlined here is similarly effective at lowering cholesterol, but also improves metabolism, insulin response, oxygen flow to the heart, brain, and body, arterial and neural flexibility, and more.

Another reason why I prescribe red yeast rice extract over statins whenever possible is that, in my observation, people on red yeast rice extract tend to have less severe and less frequent negative side effects than those on statins. Biochemically, the carbon structure of red yeast rice has a different bioactivity and bioavailability than statin drugs, and that's what makes the red yeast rice extract slightly easier on your system.

Red yeast rice extract is a powerful tool for improving vascular health, but it's also essentially an unregulated drug—another reason to ideally undertake red yeast rice therapy under a doctor's supervision. Buy only the highest-quality extract from a reputable manufacturer.

Niacin

Niacin is vitamin B3 and included in many multivitamins; it's also found in foods such as yeast, meat, grains, and milk. In high doses, it has been proven effective at lowering cholesterol. Niacin is available in a slow-release or time-release form that reduces flushing, and I often use it as part of the therapy for helping my patients lower their cholesterol without statins. I rarely use the prescription form (which should not be used if you're pregnant), because even the high-quality niacin I use in my clinic is very inexpensive, and thanks to the high quality there is significant benefit from a lower dose.

Niacin can do funny things to people. We're taught to tell people to take niacin at bedtime, but most women who take it wake up at 2:00 a.m. feeling flushed, hot, and sweaty. We tell patients to use the slow-release, 500-milligram niacin we prescribe with dinner and to prevent the flush by skipping it altogether if they have an extra glass of wine or spicy food with that meal. I have not had a complaint due to niacin in the ten years since we started our own line of supplements.

Omega-3 Fatty Acids (Fish Oil)

We've already talked about the incredible benefits of omega-3 in protecting the heart, but it does have a downside: omega-3 can also increase LDL ("bad") cholesterol levels. As with many supplements, omega-3 should be taken according to directions and monitoring of cholesterol levels should be included during therapy. Additionally, as with most supplements, the form of omega-3 most useful for your body is in food rather than in a supplement. Instead of taking a pill, it's better to get your omega-3 from eating responsibly harvested fatty fish that are low in heavy metals.

Destination Wellness

Think of collaboration with a doctor on your heart health as a continuum: at one end is the fifteen-minute doctor's visit where drugs are prescribed as quickly as possible to give the patient the feeling that they are getting value from the visit. In the middle is what I do most days in my clinic—helping women find their own solution. And at the other end of this continuum lies an emerging world of immersion health care: Destination Wellness. For such enormous health challenges as getting off drugs when your doctor says you must stay on them, healing complex chronic diseases, or finding a solution when traditional medicine and your best efforts have fallen short, the Taj Mahal of heart health programs is Destination Wellness (**www.menoclinic.com /destinationwellness**).

This ultimate type of collaboration between physician and patient is what I have found to be the most effective way to change people's lives for the better in the deepest fabric of their heart and soul. My Destination Wellness program is based in Jackson Hole, where we combine the healing atmosphere of the most beautiful place in the world, cutting-edge functional medicine at my clinic at the base of the Teton Mountains, and recreation therapy customized for the unique desires and passions of the individual. Our program, often attended by couples, lasts for an entire week and involves the full array of testing described in this chapter, as well as consultation on the evaluations by me and my nutritionist; training in cooking and shopping for optimal health; sunset meditation sessions; and recreational therapy options ranging from yoga to horseback riding, hiking in Grand Teton National Park, and fishing in the Snake River. Half of the typical day is spent optimizing your health with the help of me and my staff, and the other half is spent soaking in the medicine of the great outdoors or being pampered in a world-class spa.

Our life-changing Destination Wellness program is the health equivalent of a full-immersion foreign language program. It combines the best of functional medicine with an immersive experience that makes it far easier to clean out old habits such as smoking or eating junk food, to detox from environmental toxins, and to add new maintenance and healing activities such as meditation and optimal exercise—all with the oversight of a highly trained staff of experts. At the end of the week, we don't just send you home with a prescription; we connect you with a health coach in your home area, follow up at two weeks and at four weeks to see how the results of the program are working and advise you on how to adjust your solution to optimize it.

You probably didn't expect to see a program like this described in a heart disease prevention book, but in my practice I find that the key to heart health and vitality is to do everything you can to make your life better. If you can't come visit me in the Tetons, take a trip to Icaria or Okinawa and make it a Destination Wellness adventure of your own. Surround yourself with whatever sustains and heals your heart. Talk to the health gurus of your region. If you can't go that far, just go to your favorite place for a week and focus on the Precision, Personalized Solution you have in mind after reading this book. Afterwards, your partner, friends, and doctor will become your collaborators in your health, and when you make it clear that you are making decisions and pursuing a lifestyle designed to make you the healthiest woman you can be, and that you know more about your health than anyone else, they'll probably become your greatest fans. I know that my patients are some of the people I respect most in the world. I love nothing more than going out to lunch with an old patient who has regained her quality of life, listening to her joy and feeling her energy as she tells me her story of health since her time as my patient.

These are the women who are changing the world of medicine from the business of saving lives when health fails and soothing pain with drugs to a collaborative effort between doctors and patients to solve complex health issues by finding and fixing the root causes of disease and dysfunction. It is my sincerest hope that reading this book will help you become one of those women who inspires other women to ask the right questions, seek out what is best for their unique bodies, avoid heart disease, and live vital, beautiful lives powered by strong and healthy hearts.

Conclusion

The Challenge and the Promise

Our parents and grandparents—and the doctors of their era—were so awestruck by the incredible capabilities of drugs and surgery that they largely ignored the preventative, individualized approach to medicine. For most of a century, we've been so effective at systematically solving acute health problems that we've unintentionally sent the message "You can wait until you're sick, and then we'll cure what ails you." Well, as you now know, drugs and surgeries are not very effective at healing chronic issues like heart disease.

The problem for us as doctors is that we've led individuals like you to believe that modern medicine will save you when you get old and sick. Well, we can make your pain a little more bearable by giving you drugs to dull it, but we can't save you from heart disease if you don't take it upon yourself to play a role in your healing. We've convinced ourselves that we're at the pinnacle of medicine and that all we need to do is plug a patient's symptoms into an algorithm of bell curve data from clinical studies and write prescriptions. As an industry, we've grown fat on the profit of drugs that help some at the expense of many without meaningfully changing people's behavior for the better, and in many cases our best intentions are merely fanning the fires of chronic disease.

With this in mind, I'd like to end with a triple challenge and a promise—a challenge to you as an individual, to my fellow doctors, and to the industry, and a promise about your potential.

For you, the challenge is to realize that there is no guarantee that reducing chronic inflammation will prevent heart disease. Even if you do everything right, you can't be 100 percent sure you'll prevent heart disease, and at the same time someone who does everything wrong is not 100 percent guaranteed to get it. But if you try to do everything right, you can get darn close to preventing heart disease, and if you do everything wrong, you can elevate your risk astronomically. A better way to look at this challenge is to see it as incremental—every day and in every food and lifestyle decision you make, you either elevate or reduce your risk of heart disease. Exercise is a human right—or should be. If your workplace leaves no room for exercise, you're killing yourself by working there and the challenge is to find another job. Every time you make inflammatory food and lifestyle choices, you're tipping the needle toward suffering from heart disease; every time you make good food and lifestyle choices, you're tipping the needle away from heart disease. The challenge is to continuously move the needle in the right direction, even if on occasion it slips back the other way.

The crux of the individual challenge is to figure out which methods of disease prevention are right for you. Do you need to eliminate wheat and processed sugar entirely, or can you eat some of these foods without triggering an immune response? If necessary, enlist your doctor to help you figure it out, but don't put your doctor in charge. You make the final call on your treatment plan, not your doctor. I give a dozen or more presentations each year to groups of doctors, and as far as I can tell, doctors are more than ready to move beyond canned medicine and to learn how to help you with your challenge. We all read the same journals and watch with horror as heart disease remains the number-one killer. We know there is no one generic treatment that will prevent heart disease, so what we need to do is help our patients become empowered—to harness these tools to their advantage so they can come to us with information about their individuality.

My challenge to doctors is to make the patient-doctor relationship relevant again. Traditional doctors talk a lot about evidence-based medicine: we like to know there's evidence that our treatments will help the average person. The problem with this approach is that the evidence is skewed by the requirement that the treatment be applicable to the average person, and, other than mathematically, the average person doesn't really exist. Every patient needs a slightly different treatment plan to prevent disease, heal, and achieve optimal health.

I know there are a lot of excellent doctors out there who are frustrated with being purveyors of drugs rather than purveyors of health. I am 100 percent convinced that we can vastly reduce the occurrence of heart disease in women and that doing so will be exciting and demanding for doctors. Rather than treating a list of symptoms, we'll get to treat the unique inner workings of the individual. Changing from treating with drugs to treating with knowledge of the individual is a huge challenge, but the tools waiting at our fingertips are incredible, and it's a challenge that will make the practice of medicine far more rewarding than measuring a day by fifteen-minute patient visits and prescriptions written.

My challenge to the medical industry is to do a study on precision, personalized medicine. Compare one thousand individuals who have followed the preventative model outlined in this book, or a similar program, with one thousand patients following the pill-for-the-ill treatment model. Only then will we see the statistical benefit of individualized medicine.

Since that time has not yet arrived, the onus remains on the individual to be her own champion for individualized medicine and to shape her behavior and lifestyle to ensure a long life complete with the beauty of a healthy heart.

One key to meeting these challenges is to understand what it was like for our great-great-grandparents, who experienced preventative, individualized medicine, but without our modern capabilities. Treatments in those days were so dangerous and ineffective that their only option was to prevent disease in the first place. The doctors of their era rode around on horseback, making house calls, attending to the sick, and advising on the best practices of the day to achieve health. They'd certainly try to save a person who was sick, but more often than not, if an individual was sick, it was already too late. In those days, there were no clinical trials as we know them today. The first truly randomized, controlled clinical trial was in 1946, conducted for the antibiotic streptomycin. A few years earlier, in 1943, the first double-blind controlled study was done on patulin, a cold medication. So before then, rather than use treatments based on numbers, doctors treated based on the individual.

Medicine has come a long way in the last seventy years, but at this point, in spite of that progress, we're also suffering a collective drug-and-surgery hangover as the first century of clinical trial–based medicine draws to a close. To reach the next chapter in medicine and health, all of us—individuals, doctors, and the industry—need to meet the challenge to change. Luckily for us and for future generations, we're starting to make the needed changes. With access not only to clinical trials but to the very best cutting-edge biochemical and biophysical assessment techniques to reveal individual imbalances and inflammatory triggers and a vast body of knowledge from our deep experience with acute treatment, we're now learning how to apply all of this on an individual level.

Is it any wonder that functional medicine is the hottest game in the health industry right now? Functional medicine conferences sell out four months in advance. The luminaries in the field are on nonstop speaking tours of conferences, medical schools, hospitals, and universities and are hired as consultants for pharmaceutical companies, diagnostic laboratories, and medical centers. Instead of riding horses and carrying our tools in a leather satchel, today's traveling functional medicine doctors are riding in planes, evaluating patients by using electronic media before even meeting them, and collaborating with advanced diagnostic laboratories that make even rocket science look simple. The ultimate goal is to move beyond the last seventy years of neglecting the individual in favor of statistical diagnoses and pill-for-the-ill medicine. The tools may have changed, but we've learned that the best medicine still requires doctors to go from patient to patient, paying the same attention to the individual as if they were riding miles on horseback between house calls.

An awakening is also underway for individuals—the realization that drugs and surgery aren't nearly as effective for healing as the power of their own bodies. Just like those visited by the doctors of yesteryear after they got back on their horse and rode away, you're responsible for your own health and healing. It's up to you to heal, to reduce the unhealthy impacts on your life, and to increase the healthy influences. If you cut off your foot with an ax while chopping wood, we can do things to save your foot or even build you a new one—both medical miracles that were unimaginable a century ago. But if your lifestyle saturates your body with inflammation, even the best of today's medicine will do little to help you. In fact, to prevent disease and truly heal your heart, you might have been in better hands with the attentive doctor on horseback than today's institution of medicine, which is designed to wait until you have the disease before beginning treatment.

The heart disease that women suffer from today is an ailment of the modern woman, and to rid ourselves of this economically and individually debilitating disease, we need to take a lesson from the past while looking to the future. For the industry, billions of dollars are waiting to be made in the prevention of heart disease. For doctors, work is about to get a lot more exciting and rewarding than it has been since we last saddled up and rode hard to save someone's life. And for you, it is a time of empowerment, a time when you tell your doctor what you need and make decisions every day that will extend—not just by years but by decades—the pleasurable, vital, vibrant, active, and memorable times of your life.

I'll end with the promise: if you grab ahold of the solution we have designed together while reading this book, I promise you that your life will get better. Your risk of heart disease will decline. You will become a hero to your friends and family for your bold confidence in your ability to change your life. This is what I've seen my patients do, and I promise—you can do it too.

Appendix

7-Day Food Log

Day 1

Date:

Breakfast   Time:

_____

_____

_____

Snacks   Time:

_____

_____

_____

Lunch   Time:

_____

_____

_____

Snacks   Time:

_____

_____

_____

Dinner   Time:

_____

_____

_____

Snacks   Time:

_____

_____

_____

Beverages   Time:

_____

_____

_____

Irritability Prior to Eating?	Yes No	Energy Level: 0–10 _____
Sleepy After Eating?	Yes No	Mood: 0–10 _____
Gas or Bloating?	Yes No	Sleep: 0–10 _____
Bowel Movement?	Yes No	

Day 2

Date:

Breakfast   Time:

_____

_____

_____

Snacks   Time:

_____

_____

Lunch   Time:

_____

_____

_____

Snacks   Time:

_____

_____

Dinner   Time:

_____

_____

_____

Snacks   Time:

_____

_____

Beverages   Time:

_____

_____

_____

Irritability Prior to Eating?	Yes	No	Energy Level: 0–10 _____
Sleepy After Eating?	Yes	No	Mood: 0–10 _____
Gas or Bloating?	Yes	No	
Bowel Movement?	Yes	No	Sleep: 0–10 _____

Day 3

Date:

Breakfast | Time:

_____

_____

Snacks | Time:

_____

_____

Lunch | Time:

_____

_____

Snacks | Time:

_____

_____

Dinner | Time:

_____

_____

Snacks | Time:

_____

_____

Beverages | Time:

_____

_____

Irritability Prior to Eating?	Yes	No	Energy Level: 0–10 _____
Sleepy After Eating?	Yes	No	Mood: 0–10 _____
Gas or Bloating?	Yes	No	
Bowel Movement?	Yes	No	Sleep: 0–10 _____

Day 4

Date:

Breakfast   **Time:**

_____

_____

_____

Snacks   **Time:**

_____

_____

_____

Lunch   **Time:**

_____

_____

_____

Snacks   **Time:**

_____

_____

_____

Dinner   **Time:**

_____

_____

_____

Snacks   **Time:**

_____

_____

_____

Beverages   **Time:**

_____

_____

_____

Irritability Prior to Eating?	Yes No	Energy Level: 0–10 _____
Sleepy After Eating?	Yes No	Mood: 0–10 _____
Gas or Bloating?	Yes No	
Bowel Movement?	Yes No	Sleep: 0–10 _____

Day 5

Date:

Breakfast   Time:

_____

_____

Snacks   Time:

_____

_____

Lunch   Time:

_____

_____

Snacks   Time:

_____

_____

Dinner   Time:

_____

_____

Snacks   Time:

_____

_____

Beverages   Time:

_____

_____

Irritability Prior to Eating?	Yes	No	Energy Level: 0–10 _____
Sleepy After Eating?	Yes	No	Mood: 0–10 _____
Gas or Bloating?	Yes	No	Sleep: 0–10 _____
Bowel Movement?	Yes	No	

Day 6

Date:

Breakfast	Time:

_____

_____

Snacks	Time:

_____

_____

Lunch	Time:

_____

_____

Snacks	Time:

_____

_____

Dinner	Time:

_____

_____

Snacks	Time:

_____

_____

Beverages	Time:

_____

_____

Irritability Prior to Eating?	Yes	No	Energy Level: 0–10 _____
Sleepy After Eating?	Yes	No	Mood: 0–10 _____
Gas or Bloating?	Yes	No	
Bowel Movement?	Yes	No	Sleep: 0–10 _____

Day 7

Date:

Breakfast	**Time:**

_____

_____

Snacks	**Time:**

_____

_____

Lunch	**Time:**

_____

_____

Snacks	**Time:**

_____

_____

Dinner	**Time:**

_____

_____

Snacks	**Time:**

_____

_____

Beverages	**Time:**

_____

_____

Irritability Prior to Eating?	Yes	No
Sleepy After Eating?	Yes	No
Gas or Bloating?	Yes	No
Bowel Movement?	Yes	No

Energy Level: 0–10 _____

Mood: 0–10 _____

Sleep: 0–10 _____

Acknowledgments

Writing this book was a true labor of love and is an accumulation of over thirty-five years of study. To all my patients that I've learned from, cared for, cried with, and had care for me—you are the inspiration for what I do every day. You have opened my eyes and my heart for the need to tell the story the right way. My vision of bringing personalized care to all women, which has helped thousands of women, is inspired by you, and it is clear to me how important this work is to all of you.

Heartfelt thanks go out to the entire team at HarperOne publishing. To my editors, Sydney Rogers and Gideon Weil—I deeply appreciate how you have provided the expertise, collaborative energy, and continued momentum for carrying out this message of change for women's heart health. The passion you bring to your work and to this message has inspired me to produce a book at the highest level. To Stephanie Tade, thank you inspiring me to be the best I can, for connecting the relationships with the dream team at HarperOne. You immediately saw how important this book could be and connected us to make it happen.

We stand on the shoulders of giants who before us have lit the torch and led the way. Dr. Jeffrey Bland lit the spark of functional medicine for me twenty years ago and has always shown me the way to keep the light bright. Jeff blends the best of science with the heart of medicine and has taught me how to see patterns when I thought there were none. From all of us working in the trenches to help people daily, we deeply thank you, Jeff. To all the faculty, staff, and members at the Institute for Functional Medicine, I greatly appreciate the work that you do to teach and share the tools for the future of medicine.

This project would not have been possible without the friendship of my whole community of doctors and friends, with whom I work as a tribe of healers to make a difference every day. You are all the cocreators of our future and the transformation of chronic illness, including heart disease. All things are now possible working together. The rising tide does truly lift all boats.

This book could not have been accomplished without the energy, creativity, and passion of Topher Donahue; the wisdom of his wife, Vera; the otherworldly attention span and maturity of his twin daughter and son, Aya and Keahi; his mother, Peggy, for being a role model for women's heart health; and dear friends Laura and Raymond Farris—thank you for bringing all of us together and sharing in the magic of this message.

The team in my clinic is crucial to delivering the care we strive for: thank you to all past and present team members, as you are my second family and my success is greatly due to your efforts in providing care and love to those who visit us. Sincere thank you to Aaron Lundin, my longtime team mate in this adventure.

True knowledge is always honed by good mentors. I am blessed to have had good mentors in my life. Dean Ornish was the first who showed me what was possible using lifestyle medicine and inspired me to share with you the future of personalized medicine. I've recently had the great fortune to have a new mentor my life, Dr. Jack Stark. My father was his mentor and he has become my dear friend and passionate mentor. With him on my team I feel all things are possible.

To Lenka and Isabella, thank you for bringing joy to my life every day and for teaching me how to be in love. To my children, Anthony and Jueliet, you are the reason I wake up every day and do my part to help make the world a better place. I am so very proud of both of you and love you with all my heart.

Coming from an amazing family of six children with four doctors, including Mike, Scott, and Shelly; a genius architect, Amy; and an amazing fashion designer, Cinthia (CINO)—I thank all my brothers and sisters for helping me to become who I am. Our connection all started and was maintained by our mother, whose infectious smile to this day warms my heart as I drive down the tree-lined street to our home to see her. Ringing the dinner bell out on the deck for us to come together at the table, where we all sat and shared stories of the day, our fears of tomorrow, and our dreams of the future in a space that allowed them to come true for all of us. To my father, Frank—I wish we could have had more time together in your short but amazing life, and I am eternally thankful that I made the time to learn from you all that I could. I think of you and feel you with me daily and cherish the inspiration, passion, and compassion you have instilled in me.

And last, I want to thank you, the reader, for wanting the best for yourself and working to find a better way. My hope is that together we find the path to a healthier future for yourself and the next generation of women.

Selected Bibliography

Chapter 1

Lori Mosca, Elizabeth Barrett-Connor, and Nanette Kass Wenger, "Sex/Gender Differences in Cardiovascular Disease Prevention: What a Difference a Decade Makes," *Circulation* 124, no. 19 (November 2011): 2145–54.

A. H. Maas and Y. E. Appelman, "Gender Differences in Coronary Heart Disease," *Netherlands Heart Journal* 18, no. 11 (November 2010): 598–603.

"Physicians' Health Study," *New England Journal of Medicine* (July 20, 1989): 1825–28.

Anita Holdcroft, "Gender Bias in Research: How Does It Affect Evidence Based Medicine?," *Journal of the Royal Society of Medicine* (January 2007): 2–3.

Maria Cecilia Solimene, "Coronary Heart Disease in Women: A Challenge for the 21st Century," *Clinics* (Sao Paulo) 65, no. 1 (January 2010): 99–106.

Women's Heart Foundation, "Women and Heart Disease Facts, 2018," www.womensheart.org/content/heartdisease/heart_disease_facts .asp.

Rebecca W. Persky, Lisa Christine Turtzo, and Louise D. McCullough, "Stroke in Women: Disparities and Outcomes," *Current Cardiology Reports* 12, no. 1 (January 2010): 6–13.

S. A. Peters, R. R. Huxley, and M. Woodward, "Diabetes as Risk Factor for Incident Coronary Heart Disease in Women Compared with Men: A Systematic Review and Meta-analysis of 64 Cohorts Including 858,507 Individuals and 28,203 Coronary Events," *Diabetologia* 57, no. 8 (August 2014): 1542–51.

Alzheimer's Association, "2018 Alzheimer's Facts and Figures," www .alz.org/facts.

Edward W. Gregg, Qiuping Gu, Yiling J. Cheng, et al., "Mortality Trends in Men and Women with Diabetes, 1971 to 2000," *Annals of Internal Medicine* 147, no. 3 (August 2007): 149–55.

P. A. Mehta and M. R. Cowie, "Gender and Heart Failure: A Population Perspective," *Heart* 92, Suppl. 3 (May 2006): iii14–18.

Lynda Lisabeth and Cheryl Bushnell, "Menopause and Stroke: An Epidemiologic Review," *Lancet Neurology* 11, no. 1 (January 2012): 82–91.

Albert Oberman, Allen R. Myers, Thomas M. Karunas, et al., "Heart Size of Adults in a Natural Population—Tecumseh, Michigan," *Circulation* 35, no. 4 (April 1967): 724–33.

Jason C. Siegler, Shafiq Rehman, Geetha P. Bhumireddy, et al., "The Accuracy of the Electrocardiogram During Exercise Stress Test Based on Heart Size," *PLOS One* 6, no. 8 (August 2011): e23044.

Jaroslaw Krejza, Michal Arkuszewski, Scott E. Kasner, et al., "Carotid Artery Diameter in Men and Women and the Relation to Body and Neck Size," *Stroke* 37 (March 2006): 1103–5.

Joel Lexchin, Lisa A Bero, Benjamin Djulbegovic, et al., "Pharmaceutical Industry Sponsorship and Research Outcome and Quality: Systematic Review," *BMJ* 326, no. 7400 (May 2003): 1167.

Chapter 2

L. de Graaf, A. H. P. M. Brouwers, and W. L. Diemont, "Is Decreased Libido Associated with the Use of HMG-CoA-Reductase Inhibitors?," *British Journal of Clinical Pharmacology* 58, no. 3 (September 2004): 326–28.

G. Zuliani, M. Cavalieri, M. Galvani, et al., "Relationship Between Low Levels of High-Density Lipoprotein Cholesterol and Dementia in the Elderly: The InChianti Study," *Gerontological Society of America* 73, no. 3 (March 2018): 415–18.

Beth A. Abramovitz and Leann L. Birch, "Five-Year-Old Girls' Ideas About Dieting Are Predicted by Their Mothers' Dieting," *Journal of the American Dietetic Association* 100, no. 10 (October 2000): 1157–63.

Canadian Paediatric Society, "Dieting: Information for Teens," *Paediatrics & Child Health* 9, no. 7 (September 2004): 495–96.

Flavia Fayet, Peter Petocz, and Samir Samman, "Prevalence and Correlates of Dieting in College Women: A Cross Sectional Study," *International Journal of Women's Health* 4 (August 2012): 405–11.

S. A. French and R. W. Jeffery, "Consequences of Dieting to Lose Weight: Effects on Physical and Mental Health," *Health Psychology* 13, no. 3 (May 1994): 195–212.

I. Anderson, M. Parry-Billings, E. Newsholme, et al., "Dieting Reduces Plasma Tryptophan and Alters Brain 5-HT Function in Women," *Psychological Medicine* 20, no. 4 (1990): 785–91, https://doi.org/10.1017/S0033291700036473.

Amy Maxmen, "Calorie Restriction Falters in the Long Run," *Nature* 488, no. 7413 (August 2012): 569, https://doi.org/10.1038/488569a.

Frank B. Hu, Meir J. Stampfer, JoAnn E. Manson, et al., "Dietary Fat Intake and the Risk of Coronary Heart Disease in Women," *New England Journal of Medicine* 337 (November 1997): 1491–99, https://doi.org/10.1056/NEJM199711203372102.

Berkeley Wellness, "Ornish: Still Best for Heart Health?," January 2015, http://www.berkeleywellness.com/healthy-eating/diet-weight-loss/article/ornish-still-ultimate-diet.

Jeannette Moninger, "Andrew Weil's Anti-Inflammatory Diet," WebMD, February 2018.

C. Malo and J. X. Wilson, "Glucose Modulates Vitamin C Transport in Adult Human Small Intestinal Brush Border Membrane Vesicles," *Journal of Nutrition* 130, no. 1 (January 2000): 63–69.

Cynthia A. Daley, Amber Abbott, Patrick S. Doyle, et al., "A Review of Fatty Acid Profiles and Antioxidant Content in Grass-Fed and Grain-Fed Beef," *Nutrition Journal* 9, no. 10 (March 2010), https://doi.org/10.1186/1475-2891-9-10.

Wilfred Leith, "Experiences with the Pennington Diet in the Management of Obesity," *Canadian Medical Association Journal* 84, no. 25 (June 1961): 1411–14.

Harvard Heart Letter, "10 Myths About Heart Disease," Harvard Health Publishing, June 2013, www.health.harvard.edu/heart-health/10-myths-about-heart-disease.

Harvard Heart Letter, "Heart Attack Despite Low Cholesterol?," Harvard Health Publishing, December 2015, www.health.harvard.edu/heart-health/ask-the-doctor-heart-attack-despite-low-cholesterol.

M. L. Fernandez, "Rethinking Dietary Cholesterol," *Current Opinion in Clinical Nutrition and Metabolic Care* 15, no. 2 (March 2012): 117–21, https://doi.org/10.1097/MCO.0b013e32834d2259.

Andrew Thompson and Norman J. Temple, "The Case for Statins: Has It Really Been Made?," *Journal of the Royal Society of Medicine* 97, no. 10 (October 2004): 461–64.

Jeanne Garbarino, "Cholesterol and Controversy: Past, Present and Future," *Scientific American*, November 2001, blogs.scientific american.com/guest-blog/cholesterol-confusion-and-why-we-should -rethink-our-approach-to-statin-therapy.

Samuel Stebbins, "The World's 15 Top Selling Drugs," 24/7 Wall St., April 2016, 247wallst.com/special-report/2016/04/26/top-selling -drugs-in-the-world/2.

Mark Jones, Susan Tett, Geeske M. E. E. Peeters, et al., "New-Onset Diabetes After Statin Exposure in Elderly Women: The Australian Longitudinal Study on Women's Health," *Drugs and Aging* 34 (March 2017): 203, https://doi.org/10.1007/s40266-017-0435-0.

Harvard Health Publishing, "Gender Matters: Heart Disease Risk in Women," March 2017, www.health.harvard.edu/heart-health /gender-matters-heart-disease-risk-in-women.

Randy A. Sansone, "Cholesterol Quandaries: Relationship to Depression and the Suicidal Experience," *Psychiatry* (Edgemont) 5, no. 3 (March 2008): 22–34.

H. You, W. Lu, S. Zhao, et al., "The Relationship Between Statins and Depression: A Review of the Literature," *Expert Opinion on Pharmacotherapy* 14, no. 11 (August 2013): 1467–76, published online June 17, 2013, https://doi.org/10.1517/14656566.2013.803067.

Cassie Redlich, Michael Berk, Lana J. Williams, et al., "Statin Use and Risk of Depression: A Swedish National Cohort Study," *BMC Psychiatry* 14 (December 2014): 348.

The NNT, November 2017, www.thennt.com/nnt/statins-for-heart -disease-prevention-without-prior-heart-disease.

Umme Aiman, Ahmad Najmi, and Rahat Ali Khan, "Statin Induced Diabetes and Its Clinical Implications," *Journal of Pharmacology and Pharmacotherapeutics* 5, no. 3 (July–September 2014): 181–85.

Kevin D. Hall, Thomas Bemis, Robert Brychta, et al., "Calorie for Calorie, Dietary Fat Restriction Results in More Body Fat Loss than

Carbohydrate Restriction in People with Obesity," *Cell Metabolism* 22, no. 3 (August 2015): 427–36.

Alexander Van Tulleken, "One Twin Gave Up Sugar, the Other Gave Up Fat. Their Experiment Could Change YOUR Life," *Daily Mail*, January 2014, www.dailymail.co.uk/health/article-2546975/One -twin-gave-sugar-gave-fat-Their-experiment-change-YOUR-life.html.

D. S. Grimes, "Statins and Changing Number Needed to Treat (NNT)," *Journal of Cardiovascular Disorders* 2, no. 3 (2015): 1018.

A. L. Culver, I. S. Ockene, R. Balasubramanian, et al., "Statin Use and Risk of Diabetes Mellitus in Postmenopausal Women in the Women's Health Initiative," *Archives of Internal Medicine* 172, no. 2 (January 2012): 144–52, https://doi.org/10.1001/archinternmed.2011.625, published online January 9, 2012.

D. J. Becker, R. Y. Gordon, P. B. Morris, et al., "Simvastatin vs Therapeutic Lifestyle Changes and Supplements: Randomized Primary Prevention Trial," *Mayo Clinic Proceedings* 83, no. 7 (July 2008): 758–64, https://doi.org/10.4065/83.7.758.

Qing Yang, "Gain Weight by 'Going Diet?' Artificial Sweeteners and the Neurobiology of Sugar Cravings," *The Yale Journal of Biology and Medicine* 3, no. (June 2010): 101–8.

Sripal Bangalore, Rana Fayyad, Rachel Laskey, et al., "Body-Weight Fluctuations and Outcomes in Coronary Disease," *New England Journal of Medicine* 376 (April 2017): 1332–40, https://doi.org/10 .1056/NEJMoa1606148.

F. Taylor, K. Ward, T. H. Moore, et al., "Statins for the Primary Prevention of Cardiovascular Disease," *The Cochrane Database of Systematic Reviews* 1 (2011): CD004816, https://doi.org/10.1002 /14651858.CD004816.pub4.

K. K. Ray, S. R. Seshasai, S. Erqou, et al., "Statins and All-Cause Mortality in High-Risk Primary Prevention: A Meta-analysis of 11 Randomized Controlled Trials Involving 65,229 Participants," *Archives Internal Medicine* 170, no. 12 (June 2010): 1024–31, PubMed PMID: 20585067.

B. A. Parker, J. A. Capizzi, A. S. Grimaldi, et al., "Effect of Statins on Skeletal Muscle Function," *Circulation* 127, no. 1 (2013): 96–103.

D. D. Waters, J. E. Ho, D. A. DeMicco, et al., "Predictors of New-Onset Diabetes in Patients Treated with Atorvastatin: Results from 3 Large

Randomized Clinical Trials," *Journal of the American College of Cardiology* 57, no. 14 (2011): 1535–45.

S. Yusuf, J. Bosch, G. Dagenais, et al., "HOPE-3 Investigators: Cholesterol Lowering in Intermediate-Risk Persons Without Cardiovascular Disease," *New England Journal of Medicine* 374, no. 21 (2016): 2021–31.

F. Godlee, "Statins: We Need an Independent Review," *BMJ* 354 (September 2016): i4992, https://doi.org/10.1136/bmj.i4992.

K. Stergiopoulos, W. E. Boden, P. Hartigan, et al., "Percutaneous Coronary Intervention Outcomes in Patients with Stable Obstructive Coronary Artery Disease and Myocardial Ischemia: A Collaborative Meta-analysis of Contemporary Randomized Clinical Trials," *JAMA Internal Medicine* 174, no. 2 (2014): 232–40.

U. Aiman, A. Najmi, and R. A. Khan, "Statin Induced Diabetes and Its Clinical Implications," *Journal of Pharmacology & Pharmacotherapeutics* 5, no. 3 (2014): 181–85, https://doi.org/10.4103/0976-500X.136097.

A. Skarlovnik, M. Janić, M. Lunder, et al., "Coenzyme Q10 Supplementation Decreases Statin-Related Mild-to-Moderate Muscle Symptoms: A Randomized Clinical Study," *Medical Science Monitor: International Medical Journal of Experimental and Clinical Research* 20 (2014): 2183–88, https://doi.org/10.12659/MSM.890777.

P. Thavendiranathan, "Primary Prevention of Cardiovascular Disease with Statin Therapy," *Archives Internal Medicine* 166 (2006): 2307–13.

CTT Collaborators, "Efficacy and Safety of Cholesterol-Lowering Treatment: Prospective Meta-analysis of Data from 90,056 Participants in 14 Randomized Trials of Statins," *Lancet* 366 (2005): 1267–78.

P. M. Ridker, E. Danielson, F. A. Fonseca, et al., "Rosuvastatin to Prevent Vascular Events in Men and Women with Elevated C-reactive Protein," *New England Journal of Medicine* 359, no. 21 (2008): 2195–207.

J. M. Wright, "Do Statins Have a Role in Primary Prevention? An Update," *Therapeutics Letter* 2010, vol. 77.

J. J. Brugts, T. Yetgin, S.E. Hoeks, et al., "The Benefits of Statins in People Without Established Cardiovascular Disease but with Cardiovascular Risk Factors: Meta-analysis of Randomised Controlled Trials," *British Medical Journal* 338 (June 2009): b2376, https://doi.org/10.1136/bmj.b2376, PubMed PMID: 19567909, PubMed Central PMCID: PMC2714690.

B. A. Parker, J. A. Capizzi, A. S. Grimaldi, et al., "Effect of Statins on Skeletal Muscle Function," *Circulation* 127, no. 1 (2013): 96–103.

E. J. Mills, B. Rachlis, P. Wu, et al., "Primary Prevention of Cardiovascular Mortality and Events with Statin Treatments: A Network Meta-analysis Involving More Than 65,000 Patients," *Journal of the American College of Cardiology* 52, no. 22 (November 25, 2008): 1769–81, PubMed PMID: 19022156.

R. Chou, T. Dana, I. Blazina, et al., "Statins for the Prevention of Cardiovascular Disease in Adults: Evidence Report and Systematic Review for the U.S. Preventive Services Task Force," *JAMA* 316, no. 19 (2016): 2008–24.

J. Abramson and J. M. Wright, "Are Lipid-Lowering Guidelines Evidence-Based?," *Lancet* 369, no. 9557 (January 2007): 168–69, PubMed PMID: 17240267.

R. F. Redberg and M. H. Katz, "Statins for Primary Prevention: The Debate Is Intense, but the Data Are Weak," *JAMA* 316, no. 19 (2016): 1979–81.

J. Fulcher, R. O'Connell, M. Voysey, et al., "Cholesterol Treatment Trialists' Collaboration. Efficacy and Safety of LDL-Lowering Therapy Among Men and Women: Meta-analysis of Individual Data from 174,000 Participants in 27 Randomised Trials," *Lancet* 385, no. 9976 (2015): 1397–405.

N. Sattar, D. Preiss, H. M. Murray, et al., "Statins and Risk of Incident Diabetes: A Collaborative Meta-analysis of Randomised Statin Trials," *Lancet* 375, no. 9716 (February 27, 2010): 735–42, published online February 16, 2010, PubMed PMID: 20167359.

A. P. Agouridis, M. S. Kostapanos, and M. S. Elisaf, "Statins and Their Increased Risk of Inducing Diabetes," *Expert Opinion on Drug Safety* 14, no. 12 (2015): 1835–44, https://doi.org/10.1517/14740338.2015.1096 343, published online October 5, 2015.

B. Mihaylova, J. Emberson, L. Blackwell, et al., "Cholesterol Treatment Trialists' Collaborators. The Effects of Lowering LDL Cholesterol with Statin Therapy in People at Low Risk of Vascular Disease: Meta-analysis of Individual Data from 27 Randomised Trials," *Lancet* 380, no. 9841 (2012): 581–90.

A. L. Culver, I. S. Ockene, R. Balasubramanian, et al., "Statin Use and Risk of Diabetes Mellitus in Postmenopausal Women in the Women's Health Initiative," *Archives Internal Medicine* 172, no. 2 (January 2012): 144–52, https://doi.org/10.1001/archinternmed.2011.625, published online January 9, 2012.

D. S. Grimes, "Statins and Changing Number Needed to Treat (NNT)," *Journal of Cardiovascular Disorders* 2, no. (2015): 1018.

Chapter 3

Sheldon Cohen, Denise Janicki-Deverts, William J. Doyle, et al., "Chronic Stress, Glucocorticoid Receptor Resistance, Inflammation, and Disease Risk," *Proceedings of the National Academy of Sciences* 109, no. 16 (April 2012): 5995–99, https://doi.org/10.1073/pnas .1118355109.

H. L. Chen, T. C. Tsai, Y. C. Tsai, et al., "Kefir Peptides Prevent High-Fructose Corn Syrup–Induced Non-alcoholic Fatty Liver Disease in a Murine Model by Modulation of Inflammation and the JAK2 Signaling Pathway," *Nutrition and Diabetes* 6 (December 2016): e237, https://doi.org/10.1038/nutd.2016.49.

Peter J. Garlick, "Toxicity of Methionine in Humans," *Journal of Nutrition* 136, no. 6 (June 2006): 1722S–25S, https://doi.org/10.1093 /jn/136.6.1722S.

A. Fucic, M. Gamulin, Z. Ferencic, et al., "Environmental Exposure to Xenoestrogens and Oestrogen Related Cancers: Reproductive System, Breast, Lung, Kidney, Pancreas, and Brain," *Environmental Health* 11, Suppl. 1 (June 2012): S8, https://doi.org/10.1186/1476 -069X-11-S1-S8.

S. Özen and Ş. Darcan, "Effects of Environmental Endocrine Disruptors on Pubertal Development," *Journal of Clinical Research in Pediatric Endocrinology* 3, no. 1 (February 2011): 1–6, https://doi.org/10.4274 /jcrpe.v3i1.01.

William H. Goodson, Maria Gloria Luciani, S. Aejaz Sayeed, et al., "Activation of the mTOR Pathway by Low Levels of Xenoestrogens in Breast Epithelial Cells from High-Risk Women," *Carcinogenesis* 32, no. 11 (November 2011): 1724–33, https://doi.org/10.1093/carcin /bgr196.

J. H. O'Keefe, H. R. Patil, C. J. Lavie, et al., "Potential Adverse Cardiovascular Effects from Excessive Endurance Exercise," *Mayo*

Clinic Proceedings 87, no. 6 (June 2012): 587–95, https://doi
.org/10.1016/j.mayocp.2012.04.005.

K. J. Mukamal, M. Cushman, M. A. Mittleman, et al., "Alcohol
Consumption and Inflammatory Markers in Older Adults: The
Cardiovascular Health Study," *Atherosclerosis* 173, no. 1 (March
2004): 79–87, https://doi.org/10.1016/j.atherosclerosis.2003.10.011.

K. De Punder and L. Pruimboom, "The Dietary Intake of Wheat and
Other Cereal Grains and Their Role in Inflammation," *Nutrients* 5,
no. 3 (March 2013): 771–87, https://doi.org/10.3390/nu5030771.

Maki Ujiie, Dara L. Dickstein, Douglas A. Carlow, et al., "Blood-
Brain Barrier Permeability Precedes Senile Plaque Formation in an
Alzheimer Disease Model," *Microcirculation* 10, no. 6 (December
2003): 463–70.

M. K. Montgomery and N. Turner, "Mitochondrial Dysfunction and
Insulin Resistance: An Update," *Endocrine Connections* 4, no. 1
(December 2014): R1–15, https://doi.org/10.1530/EC-14-0092.

M. Alvehus, J. Burén, M. Sjöström, et al., "The Human Visceral Fat
Depot Has a Unique Inflammatory Profile," *Obesity* (Silver Spring)
18, no. 5 (May 2010): 879–83, https://doi.org/10.1038/oby.2010.22.

Boaz D. Rosen, Ravi Sharma, Kenneth D. Horton, et al., "Waist
Circumference Is a Strong Predictor of Regional Left Ventricular
Dysfunction in Asymptomatic Diabetic Patients: The Factor-64
Study," *Journal of the American College of Cardiology* 67, Suppl. 13
(April 2016): 1609, https://doi.org/10.1016/S0735-1097(16)31610-2.

Michael Randall, "The Physiology of Stress: Cortisol and the
Hypothalamic-Pituitary-Adrenal Axis," *Dartmouth Undergraduate
Journal of Science* (February 2011).

Chapter 4

Stephen M. Rappaport, "Genetic Factors Are Not the Major Causes of
Chronic Diseases," *PLOS One* 11, no. 4 (April 2016): e0154387, https:
//doi.org/10.1371/journal.pone.0154387.

C. Sylvia and W. Novak, *A Change of Heart: A Memoir* (New York:
Grand Central Publishing, 1998).

Paul Pearsall, *The Heart's Code: Tapping the Wisdom and Power of Our
Heart Energy* (New York: Broadway Books, 1999).

P. Hunter, "The Inflammation Theory of Disease: The Growing
Realization That Chronic Inflammation Is Crucial in Many Diseases

Opens New Avenues for Treatment," *EMBO Reports* 13, no. 11 (November 2012): 968–70, https://doi.org/10.1038/embor.2012.142.

T. M. Srinivasan, "Genetics, Epigenetics, and Pregenetics," *International Journal of Yoga* 4, no. 2 (July–December 2011): 47–48, https://doi.org/10.4103/0973–6131.85484.

L. Daxinger and E. Whitelaw, "Transgenerational Epigenetic Inheritance: More Questions than Answers," *Genome Research* 20, no. 12 (December 2010): 1623–28, https://doi.org/10.1101/gr.106138.110.

B. L. Beyerstein, "Whence Cometh the Myth That We Only Use Ten Percent of Our Brains?," in *Mind Myths: Exploring Everyday Mysteries of the Mind and Brain,* ed. S. Della Sala (Chichester, UK: John Wiley and Sons, 1999), 1–24.

J. A. Nielsen, B. A. Zielinski, M. A. Ferguson, et al., "An Evaluation of the Left-Brain vs. Right-Brain Hypothesis with Resting State Functional Connectivity Magnetic Resonance Imaging," *PLOS One* 8, no. 8 (August 2013): e71275, https://doi.org/10.1371/journal.pone.0071275.

S. M. de la Monte and J. R. Wands, "Alzheimer's Disease Is Type 3 Diabetes: Evidence Reviewed," *Journal of Diabetes Science and Technology* (online) 2, no. 6 (November 2008): 1101–13.

A. W. Campbell, "Autoimmunity and the Gut," *Autoimmune Diseases* (May 2014), article ID: 152428, https://doi.org/10.1155/2014/152428.

R. Sender, S. Fuchs, and R. Milo, "Revised Estimates for the Number of Human and Bacteria Cells in the Body," *PLOS Biology* 14, no. 8 (August 2016): e1002533, https://doi.org/10.1371/journal.pbio.1002533.

N. J. Abbott, "Inflammatory Mediators and Modulation of Blood-Brain Barrier Permeability," *Cellular and Molecular Neurobiology* 20, no. 2 (April 2000): 131–47.

David Epstein, "How an 1836 Famine Altered the Genes of Children Born Decades Later," i09, August 26, 2013, io9.gizmodo.com/how-an-1836-famine-altered-the-genes-of-children-born-d-1200001177.

Center for Genetics Education, "Fact Sheet 12: Mitochondrial Inheritance," 2018, www.genetics.edu.au/publications-and-resources/facts-sheets/fact-sheet-12-mitochondrial-inheritance.

A. Vojdani, K. M. Pollard, and A. W. Campbell, "Environmental Triggers and Autoimmunity," *Autoimmune Diseases* (December 2014), article ID: 798029, https://doi.org/10.1155/2014/798029.

Alan Gaby, "The Role of Hidden Food Allergy/Intolerance in Chronic Disease," *Alternative Medicine Review* 3, no. 2 (April 1998): 90–100.

Eric Wooltorton, "Tegaserod (Zelnorm) for Irritable Bowel Syndrome: Reports of Serious Diarrhea and Intestinal Ischemia," *Canadian Medical Association Journal* 170, no. 13 (June 2004): 1908, https://doi.org/10.1503/cmaj.1040882.

Chapter 5

R. Sotomayor-Zarate, G. Cruz, G. M. Renard, et al., "Sex Hormones and Brain Dopamine Functions," *Central Nervous System Agents in Medicinal Chemistry* 14, no. 2 (2014): 62–71.

X. Gao and H. S. Wang, "Impact of Bisphenol A on the Cardiovascular System: Epidemiological and Experimental Evidence and Molecular Mechanisms," *International Journal of Environmental Research and Public Health* 11, no. 8 (August 2014): 8399–413, https://doi.org/10.3390/ijerph110808399.

M. P. Monteiro, "Obesity Vaccines," *Human Vaccines & Immunotherapeutics* 10, no. 4 (April 2014): 887–95, https://doi.org/10.4161/hv.27537.

Richard D. Semba, Luigi Ferrucci, Benedetta Bartali, et al., "Resveratrol Levels and All-Cause Mortality in Older Community-Dwelling Adults," *JAMA Internal Medicine* 174, no. 7 (July 2014): 1077–84, https://doi.org/10.1001/jamainternmed.2014.1582.

R. Vidavalur, H. Otani, P. K. Singal, et al., "Significance of Wine and Resveratrol in Cardiovascular Disease: French Paradox Revisited," *Experimental & Clinical Cardiology* 11, no. 3 (Fall 2006): 217–25.

J. K. Pai, K. J. Mukamal, and E. B. Rimm, "Long-Term Alcohol Consumption in Relation to All-Cause and Cardiovascular Mortality Among Survivors of Myocardial Infarction: The Health Professionals Follow-up Study," *European Heart Journal* 33, no. 13 (July 2012): 1598–605, https://doi.org/10.1093/eurheartj/ehs047.

Isaac R. Whitman, Vratika Agarwal, Gregory Nah, et al., "Alcohol Abuse and Cardiac Disease," *Journal of the American College of Cardiology* 69, no. 1 (January 2017): 13–24, https://doi.org/10.1016/j.jacc.2016.10.048.

D. Coon, S. Tuffaha, J. Christensen, et al., "Plastic Surgery and Smoking: A Prospective Analysis of Incidence, Compliance, and Complications," *Plastic and Reconstructive Surgery* 131,

no. 2 (February 2013): 385–91, https://doi.org/10.1097/PRS
.0b013e318277886a.

G. A. Lamas, A. Navas-Acien, D. B. Mark, et al., "Heavy Metals,
Cardiovascular Disease, and the Unexpected Benefits of Edetate
Disodium Chelation Therapy," *Journal of the American College of
Cardiology* 67, no. 20 (May 2016): 2411–18, https://doi.org/10.1016/j
.jacc.2016.02.066.

V. Rondeau, "A Review of Epidemiologic Studies on Aluminum and
Silica in Relation to Alzheimer's Disease and Associated Disorders,"
Reviews on Environmental Health 17, no. 2 (2002): 107–21.

Ami R. Zota and Bhavna Shamasunder, "The Environmental Injustice
of Beauty: Framing Chemical Exposures from Beauty Products as
a Health Disparities Concern," *American Journal of Obstetrics &
Gynecology* 217, no. 4 (October 2017): 418.e1–6.

USFDA, "Lead in Cosmetics," November 2017, www.fda.gov/Cosmetics
/ProductsIngredients/PotentialContaminants/ucm388820.htm.

Consumer Reports, "How Much Arsenic Is in Your Rice?," November 15,
2014, www.consumerreports.org/cro/magazine/2015/01/how-much
-arsenic-is-in-your-rice/index.htm.

S. L. Bar, D. T. Holmes, and J. Frohlich, "Asymptomatic Hypothyroidism
and Statin-Induced Myopathy," *Canadian Family Physician* 53, no. 3
(March 2007): 428–31.

Barry P. Boden, Donald T. Kirkendall, and William E. Garrett,
"Concussion Incidence in Elite College Soccer Players," *The American
Journal of Sports Medicine* 26, no. 2 (March 1998): 238–41, https://doi
.org/10.1177/03635465980260021301.

DeLisa Fairweather, Sylvia Frisancho-Kiss, and Noel R. Rose,
"Sex Differences in Autoimmune Disease from a Pathological
Perspective," *The American Journal of Pathology* 173, no. 3
(September 2008): 600–609.

A. A. Alghasham, A.-R. M. A. Meki, and H. A. S. Ismail, "Association
of Blood Lead Level with Elevated Blood Pressure in Hypertensive
Patients," *International Journal of Health Sciences* 5, no. 1 (2011): 17–27.

L. N. Abhyankar, M. R. Jones, E. Guallar, et al., "Arsenic Exposure
and Hypertension: A Systematic Review," *Environmental Health
Perspectives* 120, no. 4 (2012): 494–500, https://doi.org/10.1289
/ehp.1103988.

Philippe P. Hujoel, Mark Drangsholt, Charles Spiekermanet, et al., "Periodontal Disease and Coronary Heart Disease Risk," *JAMA* 284, no. 11 (2000): 1406–10, https://doi.org/10.1001/jama.284.11.1406.

Fatih Tanriverdi, Harald Jörn Schneider, Gianluca Aimaretti, et al., "Pituitary Dysfunction After Traumatic Brain Injury: A Clinical and Pathophysiological Approach," *Endocrine Reviews* 36, no. 3 (June 2015): 305–42, https://doi.org/10.1210/er.2014–1065.

Joseph Carrington, "Using Hormones to Heal Traumatic Brain Injuries," January 2012, www.lifeextension.com/magazine/2012/1 /using-hormones-heal-traumatic-brain-injuries/page-02.

C. Rizos, M. Elisaf, and E. Liberopoulos, "Effects of Thyroid Dysfunction on Lipid Profile," *The Open Cardiovascular Medicine Journal* 5 (February 2011): 76–84, https://doi.org/10.2174/1874192401 105010076.

"Cholesterol Levels, Elevated," Wilson's Temperature Syndrome, www.wilsonssyndrome.com/ebook/signs-and-symptoms-and-how -they-made-the-list/cholesterol-levels-elevated.

S. L. Bar, D. T. Holmes, and J. Frohlich, "Asymptomatic Hypothyroidism and Statin-Induced Myopathy," *Canadian Family Physician* 53, no. 3 (March 2007): 428–31.

Precision, Personalized Assessment

UK Department of Health, "UK Chief Medical Officers' Low Risk Drinking Guidelines," 2016, assets.publishing.service.gov.uk /government/uploads/system/uploads/attachment_data/file/545937 /UK_CMOs__report.pdf.

V. J. Felitti, R. F. Anda, D. Nordenberg, et al., "Relationship of Childhood Abuse and Household Dysfunction to Many of the Leading Causes of Death in Adults. The Adverse Childhood Experiences (ACE) Study," *American Journal of Preventive Medicine* 14, no. 4 (1998): 245–58.

H. R. Vasanthi, N. ShriShriMal, and D. K. Das, "Phytochemicals from Plants to Combat Cardiovascular Disease," *Current Medicinal Chemistry* 19, no. 14 (2012): 2242–45.

V. Worthington, "Nutritional Quality of Organic Versus Conventional Fruits, Vegetables, and Grains," *Journal of Alternative and Complementary Medicine* 7, no. 2 (April 2001): 161–73.

Stanford Medicine, "Little Evidence of Health Benefits from Organic Foods, Study Finds," September 3, 2012, med.stanford.edu/news/all -news/2012/09/little-evidence-of-health-benefits-from-organic -foods-study-finds.html.

D. Srednicka-Tober, M. Barański, C. Seal, et al., "Composition Differences Between Organic and Conventional Meat: A Systematic Literature Review and Meta-analysis," *The British Journal of Nutrition* 115, no. 6 (2016): 994–1011, https://doi.org/10.1017/S0007114515005073.

USFDA, "You May Be Surprised by How Much Salt You're Eating," January 23, 2018, www.fda.gov/ForConsumers/ConsumerUpdates /ucm327369.htm.

S. Ramsay, S. Ebrahim, P. Whincup, et al., "Social Engagement and the Risk of Cardiovascular Disease Mortality: Results of a Prospective Population-Based Study of Older Men," *Annals of Epidemiology* 18, no. 6 (June 2008): 476–83, https://doi.org/10.1016/j.annepidem .2007.12.007.

A. Hajek, C. Brettschneider, T. Mallon, et al., "The Impact of Social Engagement on Health-Related Quality of Life and Depressive Symptoms in Old Age: Evidence from a Multicenter Prospective Cohort Study in Germany," *Health and Quality of Life Outcomes* 15 (July 2017): 140, https://doi.org/10.1186/s12955-017-0715-8.

J. A. Yanovski, S. Z. Yanovski, K. N. Sovik, et al., "A Prospective Study of Holiday Weight Gain," *New England Journal of Medicine* 342, no. 12 (March 2000): 861–67. https://doi.org/10.1056 /NEJM200003233421206.

B. A. Abramovitz and L. L. Birch, "Five-Year-Old Girls' Ideas About Dieting Are Predicted by Their Mothers' Dieting," *Journal of the American Dietetic Association* 100, no. 10 (October 2000): 1157–63, https://doi.org/10.1016/S0002-8223(00)00339-4.

Canadian Paediatric Society, "Dieting: Information for Teens," *Paediatrics & Child Health* 9, no. 7 (September 2004): 495–96.

F. Fayet, P. Petocz, and S. Samman, "Prevalence and Correlates of Dieting in College Women: A Cross Sectional Study," *International Journal of Women's Health* 4 (August 2012): 405–11, https://doi .org/10.2147/IJWH.S33920.

N. Sudo, Y. Chida, Y. Aiba, et al., "Postnatal Microbial Colonization Programs the Hypothalamic-Pituitary-Adrenal System for Stress Response in Mice," *The Journal of Physiology* 558, part 1 (July 2004): 263–75.

Chapter 7

Christopher R. Cole, Eugene H. Blackstone, Fredric J. Pashkow, et al., "Heart-Rate Recovery Immediately After Exercise as a Predictor of Mortality," *New England Journal of Medicine* 341 (October 1999): 1351–57, https://doi.org/10.1056/NEJM199910283411804.

Luciano F. Drager, R. Doug McEvoy, Ferran Barbe, et al., on behalf of the INCOSACT (International Collaboration of Sleep Apnea Cardiovascular Trialists), "Sleep Apnea and Cardiovascular Disease Initiative: Lessons from Recent Trials and Need for Team Science," *Circulation* 136, no. 19 (November 2017): 1840–50.

Chapter 9

Centers for Disease Control and Prevention, "Preventing Heart Disease: Healthy Living Habits," April 6, 2018, www.cdc.gov/heartdisease /healthy_living.htm.

S. S. Virani, "Statins in the Primary and Secondary Prevention of Cardiovascular Disease in Women: Facts and Myths," ed. S. A. Coulter, *Texas Heart Institute Journal* 40, no. 3 (2013): 288–89.

Centers for Disease Control and Prevention, "Be Antibiotics Aware: Smart Use, Best Care," December 15, 2017, www.cdc.gov/features /antibioticuse.

Michael Fine, "Quantifying the Impact of NSAID-Associated Adverse Events," *American Journal of Managed Care* 19, Suppl. 16 (2013): S267–72.

A. Nischal, A. Tripathi, A. Nischal, et al., "Suicide and Antidepressants: What Current Evidence Indicates," *Mens Sana Monographs* 10, no. 1 (2012): 33–44, https://doi.org/10.4103/0973-1229.87287.

G. N. Farhat and J. A. Cauley, "The Link Between Osteoporosis and Cardiovascular Disease," *Clinical Cases in Mineral and Bone Metabolism* 5, no. 1 (January–April 2008): 19–34.

Y. Xie, B. Bowe, T. Li, et al., "Risk of Death Among Users of Proton Pump Inhibitors: A Longitudinal Observational Cohort Study of United States Veterans," *BMJ Open* 7 (2017): e015735, https://doi.org /10.1136/bmjopen-2016-015735.

Index